Psychology for the MRCPsych
2nd Edition

Psychology for the MRCPsych

2nd Edition

Marcus Munafò MA (Oxon) MSc PhD CPsychol
Cancer Research UK General Practice
Research Group,
Institute of Health Sciences,
University of Oxford

A member of the Hodder Headline Group
LONDON

First published in Great Britain in 1998 by Butterworth-Heinemann.
This edition published in 2002 by Arnold, a member of the Hodder Headline Group,
338 Euston Road, London NW1 3BH

http://www.arnoldpublishers.com

Distributed in the USA by
Oxford University Press Inc.,
198 Madison Avenue, New York, NY10016
Oxford is a registered trademark of Oxford University Press

Whilst the advice and information in this book are believed to be true and accurate at the date
of going to press, neither the authors nor the publisher can accept any legal responsibility or
liability for any errors or omissions that may be made. In particular (but without limiting the
generality of the preceding disclaimer) every effort has been made to check drug dosages;
however, it is still possible that errors have been missed. Furthermore, dosage schedules are
constantly being revised and new side-effects recognised. For these reasons the reader is strongly
urged to consult the drug companies' printed instructions before administering any of the drugs
recommended in this book.

British Library Cataloguing in Publication Data
A catalogue record for this book is available from the British Library

Library of Congress Cataloging-in-Publication Data
A catalog record for this book is available from the Library of Congress

ISBN 0 340 80911 6

1 2 3 4 5 6 7 8 9 10

Commissioning Editor: Serena Bureau
Project Manager: Tim Wale
Production Controller: Martin Kerans
Production Editor: Jasmine Brown

Cover Design: Terry Griffiths

Typeset in 10/12pt Minion by Phoenix Photosetting, Chatham, Kent
Printed and bound by MPG Books Ltd, Bodmin, Cornwall

What do you think about this book? Or any other Arnold title?
Please send your comments to feedback.arnold@hodder.co.uk

Contents

Foreword to the Second Edition   vii

Introduction to the First Edition   viii

Introduction to the Second Edition   x

SECTION 1   PSYCHOLOGY   1

1   Basic psychology   3

2   Social psychology   63

3   Neuropsychology   93

4   Psychological assessment   101

SECTION 2   HUMAN DEVELOPMENT   117

5   Human development   119

Reading list   185

Bibliography   189

Index   191

Dedication

To Jim

Foreword to the Second Edition

Psychology is an essential part of psychiatric training and it is impossible to pass the MRCPsych examination without a good knowledge of the subject. This is especially true of the Part I examination in which a substantial proportion of the written paper (Individual Preferred Statements) consists of questions about psychology.

This book is an excellent introduction to psychology for trainees preparing for the MRCPsych examinations. The author, Marcus Munafò, has taught psychology on the Wessex MRCPsych Course for the last seven years. As a result, he realises how much psychiatric trainees know about psychology (not much!) and what they need for their exams. Trainees find him an excellent teacher who makes his subject enjoyable and easy to understand. All these qualities are reflected in his book.

Psychiatric trainees are not the only ones who will find this book useful. Psychology is an important part of their exams because of its relevance to clinical practice. It is equally important for trainees in other mental health professions, such as nursing, social work and occupational therapy. The book also provides a good refresher for trained professionals like me, who have forgotten much of the psychology we once learned.

Marcus Munafò's name is always the one I pencil in first when arranging the local MRCPsych Course timetable. I recommend that you put his book at the top of your list. It will give you a comprehensive introduction to psychology and, if you are planning to take the MRCPsych examination, it will help you pass.

Dr Ian Rodin
Consultant Psychiatrist
Co-ordinator of the Wessex MRCPsych Courses

Introduction to the First Edition

The disciplines of psychology and psychiatry, notwithstanding the inability of the majority of the public to distinguish the two, are surprisingly uncomfortable in each other's company. While a great deal of common ground exists, those trained in one tradition tend to be relatively ignorant of the methods and models of the other. As such, the recent increased emphasis placed on psychology as a basic science in the examination for membership of the Royal College of Psychiatrists, in particular in the Part One examination, requires a substantial amount of work on the part of the candidate in order to be adequately prepared for the examination.

The majority of candidates have little or no previous knowledge of psychology, while the breadth of material covered by the syllabus would not embarrass a first-year psychology undergraduate course. Moreover, the examination itself is an unusual one, given that the psychology undergraduate courses examine by means of essay questions, while the MRCPsych Part One examines by means of MCQs. Given these two features of the understanding of psychology required of MRCPsych candidates, the textbooks which currently exist for psychology are inadequate. While being, for the most part, highly readable, informative and well-produced books, they are designed for a student who has a substantial amount of time to devote to reading and who is to be examined by means of essay questions. This results in highly discursive books which do not allow MRCPsych candidates to extract the basic information required to familiarise themselves with the elements of the MRCPsych syllabus.

This book is designed to bridge the gap between the requirements of the MRCPsych candidate and the psychology textbooks which currently exist. It is not designed to be used in isolation, except as a reference tool or revision aid, and provides only the basic information and definitions which will allow the student to understand the scope and aims of the MRCPsych syllabus. In conjunction with a more traditional psychology textbook, the student will be able to identify more easily those sections of the syllabus which require more study, and will understand the jargon present in most psychology textbooks more readily. Hopefully this study will take place in the broader context of a series of lectures on psychology, among other subjects. The format of this book, therefore, follows the structure of the MRCPsych syllabus as closely as possible for ease of reference and in order to be used by students regardless of which specific course they follow.

It will be evident from any cursory inspection of this book that the emphasis is firmly on brevity. I regard it as unhelpful to produce yet another psychology textbook which covers in depth the material covered by others (far better than I could), in particular since nearly all MRCPsych candidates currently use the same textbook (Atkinson et al.'s *Introduction to Psychology*). This is not, therefore, a substitute for other psychology textbooks, but instead a familiarisation, reference and revision tool, occupying a position somewhere between a dictionary and a more traditional textbook. A substantial amount of independent work will still be required of the candidate, but hopefully this book will enable that work to proceed more efficiently and with a clear direction.

Marcus Munafò
August 1998

Introduction to the Second Edition

The basic science of psychology has not changed dramatically during the four years since the 1st Edition was published. Although psychology continues to expand in scope, and although new and important advances are being made at an unprecedented pace, the aspects of psychology examined in the MRCPsych Part I examination relate to the fundamentals of behavioural science, and these still hold. So why is there a need for a second edition?

The principal reason for the second edition is the introduction of a new format to the Multiple Choice Question (MCQ) Paper, with effect from Autumn 2001. Although the content of the syllabus remains unchanged, the 'stem' technique questions in the MCQ Paper have been replaced by Individual Statements, reducing the number of questions from 250 to 200. This change has, therefore, prompted the inclusion in the second edition of a large number of MCQs that have been re-written to conform to the Individual Statement format. In addition, the opportunity has also been taken to revise the text of Psychology for the MRCPsych to include, in particular, a greatly extended chapter on neuropsychology, and to take into account a few more years of experience in teaching on the MRCPsych Part I.

The result is, I hope, a more comprehensive text that still adheres to the principles of the first edition, namely to produce a revision handbook that succinctly summarises the key information required by the MRCPsych Part I syllabus in the areas of psychology and human development. The inclusion of sample MCQs and answers will, I hope, further add to the capacity of the book to assist a candidate in preparation for the examination in conjunction with the usual resources of a lecture course and more detailed psychology textbook.

Marcus Munafò
July 2002

1

Psychology

1	Basic psychology	3
2	Social psychology	63
3	Neuropsychology	93
4	Psychological assessment	101

1

Basic psychology

Learning theory	3	Motivation	40
Visual and auditory perception	13	Emotion	45
Information processing and	19	Stress	48
attention		States and levels of awareness	53
Memory	23	Basic psychology individual	58
Thought	30	statement questions	
Personality	34		

LEARNING THEORY

The association of events (or, more strictly, of the mental representation of events), which allows an understanding of what is likely to follow in any given situation, has obvious survival value. For example, two events closely linked in time and space, such as black skies and thunderstorms, readily become associated. It is no surprise that even the most structurally simple organisms exhibit this ability, which is also manifested, both consciously and unconsciously, in human behaviour. The robust and automatic nature of many of these learning processes may explain in part their role in the aetiology and maintenance of certain psychiatric disorders. In addition to the association of environmental events, an association between (the mental representation of) a response by the organism and its outcome allows the adaptation of behaviour to the environment. Habituation represents the simplest form of learning: any constant or repeated stimulus will result in habituation over time, for example a constantly presented tone will gradually decrease in perceived loudness. More complex forms of learning are based, primarily, on the formation of associations.

Classical conditioning

Classical conditioning represents a basic form of learning whereby one environmental event or stimulus becomes associated with another, so that the organism learns that one will follow the other. This is also known as Pavlovian conditioning after Ivan Pavlov (1849–1936), the Russian physiologist who, following work on salivatory reflexes in dogs, noticed that his dogs began to salivate on the appearance of the experimenter before any food had been presented. The presentation of food (unconditioned stimulus) leads to salivation (unconditioned response); if the former is paired with the conditioned stimulus (such as the presence of the experimenter), which would not normally cause salivation, then after sufficient pairings the presentation of the conditioned stimulus alone will lead to salivation (conditioned response). The automatic nature of this learning is important: it is not necessary for the association to be understood, although such awareness may facilitate learning.

Before learning:

| Unconditioned stimulus | UCS | Unconditioned response | UCR |
| e.g. food | | e.g. salivation | |

Learning:

| Conditioned stimulus + | UCS | Unconditioned response | UCR |
| e.g. food + experimenter | | e.g. salivation | |

After learning:

| Conditioned stimulus | CS | Conditioned response | CR |
| e.g. experimenter | | e.g. salivation | |

   The example given above, and most of the early research on classical conditioning, required an association to be formed between a biologically neutral CS and a biologically relevant UCS that would elicit an appropriate UCR. Subsequent research has shown that the association of biologically neutral stimuli is possible in animals as well as humans, although this is strictly not classical conditioning as it does not produce a CR. In this case the association of stimuli that occur in close temporal and/or spatial congruence, but which lack any appetitive or aversive properties, takes place.

Operant conditioning

Operant conditioning represents a more complex form of learning (although still largely automatic), where what is learned by the organism are the consequences of initially random or undirected actions. Also known as 'instrumental conditioning', associations are formed between the stimulus and the response, so that specific stimuli become more or less likely to elicit specific responses on the basis of the consequences of the response. Edward Thorndike (1874–1949) suggested that behavioural responses which lead to positive consequences become more likely to occur again (positive reinforcement), while those that lead to negative consequences being avoided also become more likely to occur again (negative reinforcement). This is known as the Law of Effect. For example, an animal may be conditioned to press a food lever since the consequence of this behaviour (i.e. food) is rewarding (positive reinforcement), or to press a lever to avoid a shock (negative reinforcement). Learning can be assessed directly by measuring the number of responses performed in a given period. It is important not to confuse negative reinforcement with punishment (see below). Reinforcement of any kind, whether positive or negative, increases the probability of the appropriate behaviour occurring, which is clearly not true in the case of punishment.

Observational learning

The observation of behaviour by one animal in another may also lead to the establishment of conditioned responses, both classical and operant. Observational (or vicarious) reinforcement, for example, may take place by the passive observation of behaviour in the animal that also experiences the actual reward. The association between the behaviour and the response still obtains, albeit vicariously. It is important for the subject to be able to remember the behaviour performed by the model and the consequences of that behaviour. The specific features of the model (i.e. animal in which the behaviour is observed) and the mode of observation will have an influence of the effectiveness of this form of learning (see below). Crucially, this form of learning will take longer than learning by direct exposure.

Cognitive learning

This represents a broad category of learning which involves a degree of awareness on the part of the subject. All of the above forms of learning may be facilitated by an awareness on the part of the subject of what is happening, but this is not a necessary condition. In other forms of learning this awareness is a necessary condition. Examples include the explicit transmission of facts (i.e. teaching) and problem-solving (or insight learning) where a situation is mentally restructured to find a solution. Social learning is a special case where the general principles of learning theory may be applied to the development of social competence, so that socially acceptable behaviour is reinforced, in the first instance by one's parents and subsequently by one's peers, society in general and so on. This will operate, initially, without conscious awareness but is later enhanced by a growing awareness on the part of the subject of the rules that underlie appropriate and inappropriate behaviour.

Extinction

If reinforcement ceases, the conditioned response (either classical or operant) gradually extinguishes. That is, the strength of the response decreases over time as a function of the features of the original reinforcement, in particular the reinforcement schedule (see below). The strength of response may be measured by the number of responses that continue without reinforcement over time. This is not the same as forgetting – it may be argued that all that is happening is that a different set of associations (i.e. non-associations) is being learned on top of the original pattern. That is, merely not presenting the CS will not result in the extinction of the CR with the mere passage of time. However, if the CS is repeatedly presented alone (i.e. *without* the UCS) then the response extinguishes. However, once a response has been extinguished, over time it may spontaneously recover, albeit in diminished strength, which has implications in the treatment of clinical disorders such as phobias, which incidentally provides evidence that extinction is not the same as forgetting (in the strict sense). Further evidence for this comes from data that suggest that extinguished associations can be *relearned* more quickly than in controls.

Reinforcement

Reinforcement may be positive or negative: if it is positive, the action becomes more likely to occur again because of the pleasant consequences of that action; if it is negative, the action becomes more likely to occur again because unpleasant consequences are avoided by that action (e.g. pressing a lever to avoid a shock). The effect of both types of reinforcement is an increase in the probability of the instrumental response (i.e. the behaviour). In the case of negative reinforcement, the response can be divided further into escape behaviour (which terminates the aversive event but does not prevent it) and avoidant behaviour (which prevents the aversive event from occurring in the first place). Negative reinforcement should be distinguished from punishment (see below) where a behaviour is made *less* likely because of the unpleasant consequences of the action.

When the reinforcement is clearly under the control of the organism, and it is seen as such, operant conditioning proceeds most quickly.

Learning processes and clinical problems

Theories of learning have proved particularly useful in understanding anxiety, panic and phobias, all of which seem to have features of conditioning and other learning processes in their aetiology and maintenance. In the case of phobias, this has also led to highly successful treatment programmes. These are based on the assumption that a phobia may develop if a neutral object is paired with a highly distressing event, through a process of classical conditioning. It is known that the more aversive a stimulus is, the fewer the number of pairings required for a conditioned response to be established. The phobia, once established, is hypothesised to be maintained by a process of operant conditioning, whereby avoidance of the phobic object is reinforced as the negative consequences of contact with the phobic object are avoided through a process of negative reinforcement. This two-stage model of the aetiology and maintenance of phobias has received substantial empirical support from both human and animal studies.

Three pathways to fear acquisition may be postulated (in decreasing order of the ease with which the fear is acquired in each case):

- Direct exposure (i.e. classical conditioning).
- Vicarious exposure.
- Instruction.

Depression has been suggested to be in certain ways similar to the learned helplessness displayed by subjects (usually animal) that have been in a situation where an aversive stimulus is unavoidable and subsequently make no attempt to escape an aversive stimulus when escape is possible. In the original experiments, dogs that would otherwise learn to escape shocks by jumping over a barrier to safety when a tone sounded were less able to do so if previously exposed to unpredictable and uncontrollable shocks. Other emotional, motivational and cognitive deficits also developed, leading to the suggestion that learned helplessness is an animal model of human depression.

Certain aspects of addictive behaviours may be described in operant conditioning terms, given that the consequences of drug use, for example, act as both positive and negative reinforcers (by elevating mood and concurrently allowing escape from an unpleasant situation or environment). This may account for the relatively high relapse rates of inpatient addiction treatment programmes, given that on release the subject returns to the environment that elicits the addictive behaviour. In addition, the action of certain drugs (e.g. heroin) as a UCS can result in the classical conditioning of an association between the UCR and environmental contingencies such as the location in which the drug is ordinarily taken, so that the location leads to a CR. However, most drugs elicit a CR that is an opponent response to that produced by the drug itself (i.e. compensating for the anticipated effect of the drug). This means that the organism needs to take more of the drug to compensate for this reaction. An additional consequence is that if the drug is taken in a *novel* context this CR does not occur and the amount of drug taken can result in an overdose.

Generalisation

Once a conditioned response has become established, a stimulus similar to the original stimulus will also elicit the conditioned response. The response will vary in strength as a function of the degree of similarity, so that the exact stimulus will elicit the strongest response with only slightly similar stimuli eliciting far weaker responses. This can be demonstrated experimentally by using a tone as the conditioned stimulus, which may be varied in frequency, or a light, which may be varied in wavelength. Clinically, this may help explain why phobias, for example, generalise to, say, all spiders.

Discrimination represents the ability to distinguish between similar but different stimuli, where one is reinforced and the other is not. The more similar the stimuli, the slower the ability to discriminate is to become established.

Secondary reinforcement

Primary reinforcers represent those which satisfy basic drives and needs (e.g. food, sex), while secondary reinforcers represent those which have become associated with primary reinforcers by a process of classical conditioning (e.g. money), so that they themselves have acquired reinforcing properties.

Incubation

If an emotional response is conditioned and occurs on presentation of a specific stimulus, that response will increase in strength following brief, repeated exposures to the stimulus. A phobia may become self-sustaining as escape from the phobic object leads to a reduction in the emotional response, which is negatively reinforcing. As such, the phobia is perpetuated.

Stimulus preparedness

Specific objects (e.g. blood, snakes) are much more likely to be the subject of phobias than others (it is very rare to encounter a kettle phobic). One explanation for this is that humans are biologically predisposed (or prepared) to react with fear to specific stimuli, so that conditioning occurs more quickly and is also more resistant to extinction in the case of such prepared stimuli. Convergent evidence comes from similar findings in rhesus monkeys and snake phobia, with the monkeys apparently displaying preparedness in the development of snake phobia. This need not necessarily undermine the two-stage learning model of the acquisition and maintenance of phobia but simply enhance it to explain the failure of the equipotentiality assumption (whereby all stimuli *should* have the same intrinsic potential to become phobic objects).

Escape and avoidance conditioning

As discussed above, the avoidance of a phobic object will lead to a (negative) reinforcement of the avoidant behaviour as the negative consequences of contact with the phobic object will be avoided. Furthermore, if the phobic object is encountered escape will result in a reduction in the fear response, which will lead to a reinforcement of escape behaviour (again, negative reinforcement). As described above, escape behaviour terminates the aversive event (in this case, fear) but does not prevent it, whereas avoidant behaviour prevents the fear from becoming established in the first place. This can be used to explain the maintenance of phobic behaviours. It may also be used to explain the extreme inactivity of some chronic pain patients with no identifiable physical pathology, where inactivity has become reinforced as it allows the avoidance of pain and distress, so that the inactivity continues even after the original pathology has resolved.

Clinical applications in treatment

If a role for learning, and in particular conditioning processes, is suggested for specific problems then it should be possible, using the principles outlined above, to treat that problem. Behavioural treatments such as these are concerned with the modification of behaviour for the benefit of the patient, rather than investigating the reasons for the behaviour existing in the first place. Patient consent is important as some elements of the treatment may be distressing (e.g. exposure to phobic objects). There is substantial experimental evidence for the efficacy of these treatment programmes, both from human and animal studies, in the treatment of fear and phobias, chronic pain, and so on.

Reciprocal inhibition

Desired behaviours may be increased in frequency by being reinforced with reward, while undesired behaviours may be reduced in frequency by being ignored or punished. Often, the desired and undesired behaviours are mutually incompatible, which facilitates the change in the desired direction. For example, in chronic-pain patients mobility may be rewarded, while inactivity or pain complaint may be ignored.

Habituation

This may be regarded as a form of counter-conditioning, whereby the successive presentation of a stimulus which elicits a response eventually leads to a decrease in the intensity of that response. Instinctive fear responses may be extinguished in this way in animals. In clinical application, systematic desensitisation requires patients to be exposed to the fear-provoking stimulus until the fear response subsides, which leads to a gradual extinction of the response. In this case it is extinction of a learned response (i.e. the fear response) that is the mechanism underlying the treatment, and is successful because the fear response is not sustainable indefinitely and eventually subsides. This may be facilitated by substituting the fear response with an incompatible one such as relaxation, following relaxation training. In this case, treatment is faster and also less distressing for the patient. It should be noted that exposure can include the patient simply imagining the phobic object, particularly in the case of severe phobias, with direct exposure taking place only after the fear response has partially extinguished over a number of sessions. Broadly, there are three methods of treatment:

- Flooding: enforced exposure.
- Desensitisation: gradual exposure.
- Modelling: vicarious exposure.

Chaining

A complex behaviour may be broken into a sequence of steps, with each step being learned separately. The entire chain of individual steps is then learned by bringing the steps together (either forwards or backwards) until the complex behaviour is performed in its entirety. Backward chaining may be more effective as the reward associated with the final links in the chain may be used to reinforce the learning of successively earlier links in the chain.

Shaping

This is similar to chaining, but is used when the desired behaviour is rare or absent and therefore unlikely to occur spontaneously. Successive approximations of the desired behaviour are reinforced stepwise, so that eventually the reinforced behaviour becomes similar to the desired behaviour.

Cueing

A cue represents the object or stimulus that elicits the conditioned behaviour in operant conditioning. In the case of the treatment of phobias the same cue (i.e. the phobic object) may be used to elicit an incompatible behaviour, such as relaxation. Alternatively, specific cues may be used to elicit specific desirable behaviours, for example in social skills training in autistic children. These may include signals that are used at appropriate moments, or contexts where the behaviour is required to occur.

Reinforcement schedules

Reinforcement may occur in a variety of temporal patterns or schedules: continuous, interval or ratio schedules.

Continuous reinforcement is a 1:1 contiguity of behaviour and reinforcement, which results in very quick learning but also rapid extinction. For example, lever pressing results in release of a food pellet on every lever press.

Interval schedules allow reinforcement on a given number of instances over a given period of time. For example, a food pellet may only be available for release once every minute, regardless of how many times the lever is pressed. This is a fixed-interval schedule. Alternatively, in a variable-interval schedule, one pellet may be available once every minute *on average*, in which case there will be occasions when more than one pellet is available in a minute. In animal studies, variable-interval schedules have been shown to produce more regular and more frequent responding than fixed-interval schedules.

Ratio schedules offer reward after a given number of responses (e.g. lever pressing). Fixed-ratio reinforcement is reinforcement of the behaviour only after a certain number of instances (e.g. once every four lever presses). In this case learning is slower but more robust, as extinction is also slower. Variable-ratio reinforcement is essentially a random pairing of reinforcement with behaviour at an above chance level, so that a relationship exists but is not a predictable one. That is, reinforcement is offered *on average* once every four lever presses. Here learning is slowest and, correspondingly, this reinforcement schedule is associated with the slowest extinction rate.

Punishment

Briefly, punishment represents the inhibition of unwanted behaviours by the association of the behaviour with an unpleasant consequence. This may be by the presentation of an aversive stimulus, such as a shock, on the occurrence of the behaviour, or by the omission of a desirable stimulus, such as food. In each case the behaviour being punished becomes less likely to occur in order to avoid the consequences. This may be regarded as a special case of negative reinforcement, where non-behaviour is being negatively reinforced.

Optimal conditions for observational learning

Observational learning can be regarded as a combination of classical and operant conditioning (above) and may take one of two forms: symbolic modelling (e.g. watching a video) or live modelling (e.g. watching a live actor). The latter may involve active participation on the part of the subject or may simply require observation. Furthermore, in the latter case the model may be unknown or well known to the subject. Symbolic modelling leads to the slowest learning, with live modelling being more effective. Active participation also markedly increases the effectiveness of the learning process, while the familiarity of the model also plays improves learning. Further evidence for this last effect comes from rhesus monkeys, which have been shown to develop phobias from the observation of the mother's behaviour when in contact with snakes. Note that, as in many examples given here, conscious awareness of the fact that learning is required, or that an association exists, may facilitate learning but is not a necessary condition.

Summary

- Be aware of the various forms that learning takes (classical conditioning, operant conditioning, observational learning, cognitive learning). While these have certain important features in common, there are in fact more differences than similarities, and learning should be considered in terms of its global function (i.e. adaptation to an environment) rather than more specific functions (e.g. association of events) that may only be relevant in some forms of learning. Note that some forms of learning may (or may not) be unconscious – this is relevant in the case of the development of specific clinical problems.

- Certain key definitions include extinction and reinforcement, which are related concepts. It is important to realise that extinction is not necessarily the same as forgetting, and may instead reflect the learning of a new set of contingencies that supersede previously learned associations. In the case of reinforcement, be clear on the distinction between negative reinforcement (i.e. behaviour increasing in frequency because it leads to the avoidance of negative consequences) and punishment (i.e. suppression of behaviour by pairing this with an aversive stimulus – a special case of negative reinforcement of non-behaviour).

- The aetiology and maintenance of certain clinical problems may be explained in part with reference to models of learning, in particular automatic and unconscious learning (e.g. classical and operant conditioning). Phobias, depressive illness, addictive behaviour, anxiety and panic disorders may all have features that are amenable to description with reference to learning theory. Again, there are certain key definitions that are important: generalisation, incubation and preparedness. Also be aware of the distinction between primary reinforcers and secondary reinforcers (i.e. those which have become associated with primary reinforcers).

- Given the application of learning theory in understanding the aetiology and maintenance of certain clinical problems, the next step is to be aware of the application of learning theory in treatment. The common treatment method involves habituation of some form (i.e. in varying degrees of directness), in particular in the treatment of phobias. Be aware of the distinction between chaining and shaping. The role of various reinforcement schedules is also important, in particular the influence of these on ease and rate of extinction of behaviour.

VISUAL AND AUDITORY PERCEPTION

Basic principles

The amount of information received via the various sense organs by an individual is vast and constantly changing; in order to be able to make sense of this pattern of information some degree of order must be established. In this respect, it is useful to distinguish between sensation and perception. The latter refers to the end product of a series of processes which convert the unordered information provided by the senses into meaningful and useful subjective experience, while the former simply represents the crude, unordered response elicited by external activity. The majority of research in the area of perception has been conducted on vision and hearing, and results from one area tend to be generalisable to the other, certainly in the case of general principles concerning the organisation of information into ordered units and the allocation of meaning to these units. When one considers the amount of variation possible in the information provided by the visual and auditory environments (such as variation in wavelengths reflected off an object as a function of the wavelength of the incident light) it is in fact quite surprising that the *perception* that results remains more or less constant.

Related to these abilities is the role of learning: to be able to separate an object from its background requires, in part, an awareness that it does in fact represent a distinct object. Perception is a developmental process and the nature of this development in infancy provides certain insights into the functioning of the adult perceptual systems.

Furthermore, perception is a constructive process: gaps and omissions in the information with which we are presented are completed as a result of expectations, learning processes and other cues. For example, visual depth perception relies as much on perspective and occlusion as on binocular vision and stereopsis.

Figure ground differentiation

In a stimulus containing distinct regions, we usually perceive this as one figure and the rest as ground or background. The figure stands out as clear and well-defined, while the ground is less distinct and subjectively less important. In order to be able to make out detail in specific objects we must be able to separate these objects from their background in this way. This takes place largely automatically in the early stages of the processing of visual field information. This elementary form of perceptual organisation allows attention to be focused on specific objects. It should be noted that this effect exists in other senses also: sounds may be differentiated and isolated against a general background of noise.

Object constancy

The retinal image of various objects may change widely as relative location, distance and so on vary. Regardless of this, we continue to perceive the same object, with constant shape, size and colour. There are several types of visual object constancy: shape, location, size, lightness and colour.

Shape constancy, as highlighted above, refers to the ability to the ability to perceive an object as being of a particular shape even as the retinal image changes. *Location constancy* allows successive retinal images to be associated even as the relative position of the observer and the object changes, requiring the visual system to account for both one's own movement and the movement of the retinal image. *Size constancy* enables us to perceive an object as being of a constant size regardless of its distance. In general, as an object recedes it is not seen as decreasing in size; instead it is seen as increasing in separation from ourselves, although the change in the retinal image is consistent with both interpretations. Moving an object from close to the face to three feet away results in no apparent change in size even though the retinal image is half the size. This apparently banal observation belies the substantial processing required that underlies this perceptual process. Finally, *lightness* and *colour constancies*, both related concepts, enable us to perceive objects as being of the same apparent lightness and colour as the lighting conditions, such as the wavelength and intensity of the incident light, change. Objects appear the same colour at sunset, for example, even though proportionally there is far more red light in the sunlight.

Set

In general, this refers to the tendency of organisms to respond in a stereotypical fashion to certain stimuli; in other words, it represents a cognitive readiness to react to an expected stimulus. For example, a subject used to the presentation of visual stimuli may not correctly perceive an unexpected auditory stimulus. The threshold for the perception of expected stimuli is reduced, while ambiguous stimuli tend to be interpreted in a manner congruent with expectations. These expectations will be a function of learning, past experience, and so on. Personality is one such factor in determining perceptual set, with introverted individuals being better able than extraverted individuals to sustain attention for long periods when searching a visual display for a stimulus. This has a certain clinical application, with evidence suggesting that anxious individuals react more quickly to the presentation of threatening material compared to non-threatening material, suggesting that a selective search for anxiety-congruent material occurs when anxiety is high. Such threat-related material also selectively interferes with performance on a neutral task relative to neutral material.

Other aspects

There are other features of perceptual organisation worthy of mention: the phenomenon of perceptual grouping refers to the ability to perceive a collection of dots, for example, as rows, columns, diagonals and so on, depending on our choice of grouping. The stimulus is identical in each case, but the perception quite different as a result of the chosen grouping.

Proximity also influences the perception of sensory information: two tones close together, with a pause and then two further tones will be perceived as a rhythm.

Similarity is another influence on our perception of visual and auditory stimuli: stimuli which are similar tend to be associated and grouped together, being separated from stimuli which are dissimilar.

In the case of the visual system, there is a clear tendency to prefer smooth, continuous contours, so that two curved, crossing lines will be perceived as just that, rather than four lines meeting at a point, or two sharply angled lines.

Finally, again in the case of the visual system, gaps in visual stimuli tend to be completed, so that subjective contours are the result (e.g. the Kanizsa triangle).

Many of these observations were made by Gestaltist psychologists in the 1920s and 1930s, who emphasised the role of the whole rather than the constituent parts of the perception. Although it is now acknowledged that the Gestalt school merely offered descriptions of perceptual phenomena, rather than genuine explanations, it is also true that perceptual psychologists are still fascinated by the role of the perceptual phenomena they identified.

Active perception

This is related to the work of J.J. Gibson (1904–1980), who argued that the interaction between the individual and the world produces perceptual information in itself which is not provided by the mere observation of static visual information. For example, the pattern of flow in the visual field can give us information about the direction in which we are travelling. The point towards which one is headed appears motionless, while every other point appears to be moving away from that fixed point. The speed at which these points move gives information about acceleration, deceleration, proximity, and so on. This model of direct perception bypasses the requirement that sensory information be processed in some way. However, it does not take into account the complex processing that underlies visual perception, or the role of learning and memory in the ascription of meaning to visual information.

Nevertheless, Gibson's approach emphasises that the process of moving through the world provides information in itself. For example, the visual information gained by moving laterally through a location is similar to that provided by having two eyes set a distance apart. This in turn gives depth information: hunting animals tend to move their heads from side to side when searching for prey for this reason, while military surveillance aircraft use a similar principle of stereoscopic vision, superimposing the images of two cameras set slightly apart.

A typically Gibsonian example would be an experiment where lights are affixed to the joints of an individual. If the only information available is from these lights set against a dark background, the static pattern is meaningless. If, however, the individual moves across the perceptual field, so that a pattern of motion becomes detectable among the points of light, a subject is able to determine not only that it is a person walking but also give, with reasonable accuracy, estimates of the sex and age of the actor, simply from the pattern of movement generated by the points of light.

Illusions, hallucinations and other psychopathology

Disorders of perception may take several forms. Sensory distortions represent changes in the quality, form or intensity of perceptions (either visual or auditory). For example, manic patients may display hyperacusis, i.e. increased perceptual acuity.

Hallucinations refer to perceptions (again, either visual or auditory) which are not related to any external stimuli, i.e. they are internally generated but perceived as existing externally. These are regarded by the individual as normal perceptions, and appear as 'real', not being subject to conscious manipulation (in the same way that real perceptions cannot be mentally manipulated).

Illusions, on the other hand, refer to real objects the perception of which is distorted. Dark shadows cast by bushes, for example, may be perceived as an assailant lurking. It is important to note that this is also a feature of normal perception, and the point at which this becomes pathological is important to delineate. Most people are aware of the sensation of seeing an apparently threatening shape lurking in the dark only to realise subsequently that it is, in fact, an inanimate object. Illusions tend to be more transient in nature than hallucinations, and have a strong emotional component.

Given the role of learning in processes of object identification and recognition, there may be some scope for understanding, for example, how innocuous stimuli come to be interpreted in a (usually) threatening way in some disorders.

Constitutional–environmental interaction

Neonates do not possess fully developed perceptual systems. The majority of research into perceptual development has been conducted on visual perception, with evidence that the development of the visual system is heavily dependent on interaction with the environment. If this level of interaction is reduced, for example by placing opaque goggles on infant kittens and chimpanzees, subsequent visual inadequacies are the result. For example, if the infant animal is placed in an environment consisting of only vertical stripes early in development, and if head movement is also restricted so that the only information reaching the visual cortex is of vertical patterns, the ability to perceive horizontal features is seriously impaired when the animal is later removed from this environment. If the animal is left in such an environment for a sufficient period, this impairment is permanent.

The visual cortex displays great plasticity in early infancy, so that these results are reversible if the conditions that led to them are not continued for very long. The extent to which children mimic the action of adults illustrates the importance of interaction in the development of perception. Infants prefer complex stimuli, and this effect increases with age as discrimination gradually improves. At birth, the human infant can fix, track and scan objects and shows figure–ground differentiation. These are the basic tools that allow interaction with the environment and the subsequent development of abilities such as perceptual constancies (above) and object completion (when an object is partially obscured).

Summary

- Much research into perception has been in the modality of vision (as opposed to hearing, olfaction, etc.). Nevertheless, broadly similar general principles apply across modalities, and it is often easiest to conceive of visual examples. Note also that sensation and perception are related but distinct concepts, with the latter referring to the final product of a series of computational processes that extract information of a high order from the crude data gained via the senses. An example of this is the perception of depth gained from a two-dimensional retinal image. Certain principles about our environment allow inferences to be made (e.g. in the case of depth perception, objects decrease in size with distance).
- A number of basic principles should be clearly understood: figure–ground differentiation, object constancy, and set. These are the basic tools that drive perception and allow initial crude data to be refined and additional information inferred. As such, these principles are realised in the early stages of information processing, allowing later processes to operate on the information extracted in early processing. For example, given the above cue to depth (objects decrease in size with increased distance), the ability to discriminate objects from ground is a prerequisite.

- Active perception should be regarded as an approach, rather than a specific theory. The central tenet of this is that the observer and the environment interact in a way that generates information. If one walks forward, the visual field flows in a specific way. The direction of flow gives information about the direction of travel, while the rate of flow gives information about the speed of travel. Artificially manipulating the visual field in this way can give a strong sensation of movement in stationary subjects and result in marked disorientation. Balance depends to a great extent on visual flow information feedback, so that adjustments are made to compensate for movement in the visual field. It has been suggested that this is more important in the maintenance of balance than the vestibular system.
- There are certain applications of theories of perception to clinical problems: schizophrenia and mania are the two cases where distortions of perception are common. Anxious and depressed subjects also display a tendency to detect preferentially any threatening or negative material, although this is a feature of later information processing rather than perception. The distinction between hallucinations and illusions is important.

INFORMATION PROCESSING AND ATTENTION

Information processing

It is important to realise that information refers to any input, whether tactile, visual, auditory, etc. It is best regarded rather broadly, as any material with content. Processing, then, refers to any action or function carried out on this information – for example, visual information (i.e. the retinal image) is processed to provide derivative information about depth, contour and so on, with further processing giving information about likely impending events, apparent threat and other higher-order items of knowledge.

Information processing is not necessarily conscious – indeed, the majority of information processing probably occurs automatically. Crude behavioural responses will require a degree of information processing of, say, visual material, via distinct stages of organisation, interpretation and response. This concept of progress in stages is important, and can be seen in the use of flow charts, for example, to map the pattern of information processing in any given context. This 'black box' modelling of information processing, while clearly an oversimplification, does emphasise the stages necessary for incident information to be transformed into a meaningful representation that corresponds to the subjective experience derived from this information. What is then required is an understanding of the mechanisms that operate within these black boxes, in particular the neural substrates in which these processes occur.

Attention

A common theme of psychology is the extent to which the brain is parsimonious in allocating resources. This is most clearly seen in the case of information processing and attention – given the sheer quantity of information that is present at any given time it would be impractical to process all of this to as full an extent as possible. Instead what is required is some degree of selection in the early stages of processing so that only highly salient or relevant material is processed and acted upon. This is the most frequently used meaning of the term 'attention', within which there is the further distinction of focused attention and divided attention. There are two methods that are commonly used to investigate these forms of attention:

- Focused attention tasks require subjects to attend solely to one source of information, usually whilst being distracted by another source. For example, in a dichotic listening task, different word strings may be presented from each headphone and the subject is required to attend to those from one headphone only.
- Divided attention tasks require the subject to attend to two or more sources of information simultaneously. Commonly, interference is the result of divided attention tasks, with performance on both tasks being poorer than normal. This is the case even when the nature of the two simultaneously performed tasks is quite different (e.g. visual and auditory).

Some work has been carried out on sustained attention, where the subject is required to focus, without distraction, for long periods on a single task. While there is evidence for individual differences in the ability to sustain attention for long periods, related to personality factors such as introversion, this area has attracted relatively little research.

This all assumes that there is a single entity that is 'attention', whereas in reality that which requires attentional resources will draw on several mechanisms that are likely to be related but distinct. For example, the process of shifting attention *away* from one task and the process of shifting attention *to* another task may well be distinct processes.

Models of attention (auditory)

Experimental paradigms such as those identified above have allowed the development of models that describe the relationship between incoming information and subsequent responses. Research has been carried out on both auditory and visual material. In the case of auditory material, two alternative perspectives exist.

Early filtering models argue that information is processed initially at a pre-attentive stage, with only simple features such as pitch being identified. All information needs to pass through this filter before it can be processed further. Depending on the features that are currently being attended for, some information will pass and other information will be filtered and not processed further. The majority of information, then, is lost at this pre-attentive stage of processing. Unfortunately, this model has difficulty accounting for certain well-established attentional phenomena, in particular the ability of subjects to identify highly salient material, such as their own name, in a dichotic listening task (the 'cocktail party effect'). One modification of the model that would allow for this would be for the filter to be regarded as an attenuating, rather than a blocking filter. In this way the strength of the majority of the information signal is reduced, but not eliminated altogether. The model also has difficulty accounting for the fact that visual material presented during an auditory task is well remembered, while additional auditory material is not, suggesting that parallel input can be processed effectively if they are sufficiently dissimilar.

An alternative model, also developed to account for attentional effects such as awareness of highly salient material, is the *late filtering model.* In this model, all information is processed to an equal degree in parallel. Filtering only takes place after this processing is complete, at the stage where a cognitive or behavioural response is required. One question that then arises is why we have the subjective impression of not processing a large proportion of the information we constantly receive.

It should be realised that these two types of model are not necessarily exclusive, and which is appropriate may depend on the specific demands of the situation as well as, possibly, individual differences. Certainly the modification of the early filtering model so that initial processing consists of attenuation rather than absolute filtering resolves many of the apparent difficulties, and the evidence would suggest a certain flexibility in the operation of the attentional system.

Models of attention (visual)

The findings in areas of auditory attention are also broadly generalisable to visual attention. In the latter case, however, the extent to which both early and late filtering processes occur is more apparent. The balance between these two processes depends on both automatic and voluntary processes: the attentional focus of a subject may be readily altered by concentrating on a specific stimulus, or by searching for particular information; at the same time, anxious subjects, for example, are far more easily distracted by threat material than controls, suggesting that pre-attentive, early filtering occurs even when the subject is consciously concentrating on a specific task. This only occurs, however, when there is competition for attentional resources (i.e. when there is a distractor present). When only one attentional task exists it is possible to voluntarily and strategically direct attention as required.

All sensory information, then, is processed to an equal degree pre-attentively, where simple properties are analysed. Information then passes into conscious processing, where voluntary control on the selection of material and nature of processing is far greater. One of the elements where a degree of control exists is the extent of filtering at the pre-attentive stage. In some respects focused visual attention can be likened to a spotlight that can be directed and focused as required on a relatively broad or narrow area of the visual field. Nevertheless, information that falls outside this focus may still be processed.

Information processing and schizophrenia

Attempts have been made to apply the experimental paradigms described above to schizophrenic populations. Given the models of filtering proposed, it is appealing to regard the apparent lack of filtering in the thought patterns of schizophrenics as potentially resulting from differences in the attentional systems of these subjects. Some experimental work supports this position, for example with the finding that schizophrenics are more easily distracted in dichotic listening tasks. The cognitive distortions found in schizophrenic patients may be the result of a relative lack of early filtering and a consequent overload of the late stage processing. It has also been suggested that the delusions suffered by schizophrenics are falsely interpreted as being a result of external control because the attentional system that monitors the link between the individual's intentions and actions is faulty. This system, which identifies the link between thoughts and actions, normally operates automatically at a preconscious level.

Summary

- An understanding of what information processing actually is, is important; it may be defined as any function carried out on any input or data. Sensory data, for example, is crude and unordered, and needs to be processed before any information can be derived from it. Early processing provides rough information, allowing later, more complex processing to proceed. The majority of this processing is unconscious. Information processing should be distinguished from attention, which serves to allocate limited information processing resources. Being unable to process all information fully, the brain must be parsimonious, so that learned associations allow assumptions to be made, short cuts taken, and so on.

- As in the case of theories of perception, the general principles of attention can apply to both auditory and visual attention. Information processing in the two modalities appears to be partly dissociated, so that simultaneous presentation of two sets of auditory information will result in interference, while presentation of auditory and visual information simultaneously does not result in the same degree of interference. The extent to which simultaneous presentation of information in two modalities results in interference depends on the degree to which the material presented is related (e.g. colour words, both spoken and visually presented).

- In the case of schizophrenic subjects it has been suggested that the speech and thought patterns that may characterise this condition may be explained with reference to filtering models of attention. That is, differences in the attentional systems of these subjects results in an apparent lack of filtering. There is also evidence for individual differences in attentional focus, with anxious subjects tending to search for threat-congruent material, detecting such stimuli more quickly than controls. This has been suggested as a maintenance factor in anxiety disorders.

MEMORY *Baddeley*

An initial distinction to be made is between short-term memory (STM), which resides in a short-term store (STS), and long-term memory (LTM), which resides in a long-term store (LTS). The STS can hold information for only a few seconds before it has to be consolidated in the LTS – note that this use of STS/STM is therefore quite different in psychology compared to psychiatry, where short-term memory may refer to memories held for several minutes. This distinction is inherited from early models of memory (e.g. Atkinson and Shiffrin) that suggested that information entered the STS as a necessary stage before it could be consolidated into the LTS. In this model, information initially enters a sensory store, specific to the modality of the sensory information (visual, auditory, etc.), which holds it very briefly, essentially unprocessed. This then passes to the STS, which has a very limited capacity and can hold information for a few seconds, with decay beginning immediately after the information enters. This retention may continue for longer via rehearsal (e.g. repeating words internally).

STS
↓
LTS

Transfer to the LTS begins immediately when information enters the STS, and strengthens as this transfer continues. This information may, if it remains in the STS for long enough, be consolidated in the LTS, which has a very large capacity and can store information indefinitely.

Short-term memory is also known as 'primary' or 'working' memory, while long-term memory is also known as 'secondary' memory.

Short-term and long-term stores seem to have quite different properties beyond simply the duration for which memories can be maintained in them. The STS is of a far more limited capacity than the LTS, the former being described by Milner as being able to hold '7, plus or minus 2' items of information. LTS does not appear to have any such limitation, although this is clearly difficult to confirm. Much evidence for the dissociation of the STS and LTS comes from brain-damaged patients, where either the STS is intact but the long-term memory is impaired, or conversely the STS is impaired and no new information can be consolidated in the LTS, even though long-term memories from prior to the brain damage are unaffected.

Encoding, storage and retrieval

Encoding, also referred to as registration, refers to the process whereby information is received and initially assimilated. It is therefore closely related to concepts of early information processing and attention. The extent of this initial processing in the STS is greater and more varied than might be expected, and depends on the characteristics of the material and the characteristics of the individual. An unknown language will be coded as sounds (phonemically), while one familiar with the language will code it as syntactic and semantic elements, extracting meaning from the sounds. This information processing is incorporated into models of working memory (below), which emphasises the role of the STS as an active information processing system, rather than simply a passive buffer. Memory for items in word lists is best for the first and last items on the list (primacy and recency effects, respectively). The recency effect is likely to be due to material still remaining in the STS, while the greater length of time the first material has had to be consolidated into the LTS accounts for the primacy effect. Deeper processing also facilitates consolidation to the LTS – semantic meaning is more readily consolidated than, say, phonemic content alone. This has led to the 'Levels of Processing' approach, whereby durability of memory is suggested to be a function of depth of processing. However, since the only indicator of this depth of processing is the strength of the memory trace (i.e. retrieval) the argument risks becoming circular.

Unless a rehearsal strategy is employed, storage in the STS is limited to no more than 30 seconds, with a capacity of around seven units. Most discussions of storage usually refer to the long-term store, which is of (theoretically) unlimited capacity and permanent. Some loss of information may occur, but this is slow and difficult, experimentally, to distinguish from material that remains stored but cannot be retrieved. Most 'forgetting' is in fact likely to be due to deficiencies in retrieval (see below). The organisation of LTM is described in more detail below. Material takes some time to be consolidated from the STS to the LTS, and must remain in the LTS for some minutes to be completely consolidated. Disruption of this (for example, by electroconvulsive therapy) interrupts this process and results in some degree of retrograde amnesia.

The process of retrieval is that of returning material from the LTS to STM. This is not necessarily the same as recall: the phenomenon whereby one knows that an item is known, but cannot recall it explicitly suggests some degree of retrieval (the 'tip-of-the-tongue' phenomenon), whereas recall requires conscious awareness and explicit recollection. Recognition of objects suggests that storage has taken place, but again explicit recall is not necessary. Mnemonic devices, such as associating acronyms or images with words, appear to facilitate retrieval. In general, retrieval is easier if cues exist to prompt recall; this is related to context-dependent learning, where recall of learned word lists is best in the same conditions as initial learning took place. Of course, much retrieval is implicit and occurs unconsciously, since social behaviour, object recognition and so on all require information held in the LTS to be accessed, even if the individual is not consciously aware that this process is taking place.

Working memory

Working memory refers to an elaborated model of the STS developed by Baddeley, which primarily suggests that the STS consists of several interacting subsystems, overseen by a central executive which controls these. This model integrates attention and initial processing with short-term storage, with the different subsystems representing stores for material of different modalities. For example, an articulatory loop is hypothesised to process phonological material and a visuospatial scratch pad is hypothesised to process visual material. The rehearsal of auditory material in order to maintain information in the STS for longer than 30 seconds amounts to a repeated transfer between the articulatory loop and the central executive.

Chunking

The limited capacity of the STS to approximately seven items can be extended to some degree by chunking. This is the process where several items are grouped perceptually or cognitively into larger, single units. Therefore, a string of words may be remembered by constructing acronyms for groups of the words, so that the overall number of items remains no more than seven. Similarly, the string 10-25-36-40 is easier to remember than the string 1-0-2-5-3-6-4-0.

Organisation of long-term memory

The organisation of long-term memory is complex and still far from being fully understood. Memories held in the LTS may be explicit (i.e. the individual is able to describe them completely), or implicit (i.e. the memory is apparent from behaviour rather than conscious recollection). Three types of memory should initially be distinguished:

- *Semantic memory* refers to memory for meanings, and may be described as 'knowing that', as opposed to 'knowing how'. This is related to an alternative characterisation of LTM into declarative and procedural: in this sense semantic memory is a type of declarative memory.
- *Episodic memory* is another type of declarative memory, where the memory can be explicitly recalled and described; this is memory for places, events and so on. Memories for these episodes tend to be fairly sharp and clearly delineated.
- *Procedural memory* is quite different to both types of declarative memory in that it is often difficult, or even impossible, to recall explicitly. Memories of this type include knowledge of, for example, how to ride a bike. The series of steps required to perform this act may not be explicitly known to the individual, but the action may nevertheless be performed, suggesting a rather different, implicit form of memory. Another interesting example is language, which is performed according to a set of grammatical rules which most individuals would not be able to articulate and yet which they clearly follow in that they speak (more or less) grammatically.

The organisation of items within, say, semantic memory is an area of debate, in particular whether or not items of knowledge are organised hierarchically.

Forgetting

As discussed above, the majority of supposed forgetting in the case of material held in the LTS is in fact likely to be due to a failure at the stage of retrieval. Conversely, genuine forgetting in terms of decay of the strength of the memory trace occurs rapidly for items held solely in the STS. There are, however, two theories of forgetting regarding items held in the LTS:

- *Decay theory* suggests that memories spontaneously fade over time. This is difficult to demonstrate, not least because of problems of differentiating true forgetting from retrieval deficits.
- *Interference theory* suggests that learning a second item between learning the first item and the recall of the first item impairs this recall. This may be due to impaired consolidation of the first item. Previous learning also impairs subsequent learning.

Some have hypothesised the existence of motivated forgetting (repression) but this, again, is difficult to demonstrate experimentally. In the case of the extinction of conditioned responses it has been suggested that new associations are learned which overwrite existing associations, so that when two previously associated stimuli are no longer linked this in itself is learned as a new (non-) association. Evidence in support of this position includes the spontaneous return of learned associations following extinction, and the relative ease with which an extinguished association may be re-learned.

Retrieval and emotion

Individual differences in attentional focus are known to be related to both normal and clinical anxiety; in the case of memory and retrieval there is also evidence that individual differences exist as a function of affective state, in particular depressed mood (again, both normal and clinical). Depressed subjects spontaneously recall more negative personal events and, when presented with word lists to remember, will recall proportionally more negative words from the list compared to normal controls. The difference between normal and depressed subjects is not a function of differences in motivation or overall recall, since the number of words recalled is the same in both groups. Rather it is the *quality* of the words recalled that differs, with a bias being shown towards affectively negative material in the case of depressed subjects. This is related to cognitive models of depression (e.g. Beck), which suggests that these biases in recall found in depressed subjects are in part responsible for the maintenance of the depressed state, being part of a 'vicious cycle' whereby spontaneous recall of negative material exacerbates the depressed state further.

Retrieval and schemata

Schemata refer to mental representations that allow the organisation of items of knowledge held in the LTS into related groups (e.g. animals, self-image). This accounts for the extent to which a specific event may facilitate the recall of other events, which will be related to a greater or lesser degree in the individual's personal knowledge structure. Early theories suggested a logical structure of hierarchical networks to items in semantic memory, but this failed to account for certain phenomena, for example that subjects take longer to confirm the statement 'A chicken is a bird' than they do 'A robin is a bird'. Subsequent theories placed more emphasis on organisation according to semantic relatedness, with the activation of a particular node leading to activation of related nodes (spreading activation theory). The closer the two items are in the network, the greater the extent to which one will facilitate recall of the other. These schemata also exist as patterns for behaviours in particular contexts (scripts), such as the set of rules that exist for behaviour in a restaurant, where broadly similar actions are applicable regardless of the specific characteristics of the restaurant. Finally, these schemata allow for reconstructive memory – subjects will spontaneously fill gaps in memory on the basis of the relevant schema. For example, if a passage omits certain expected actions, such as paying for tickets in a cinema, these actions are likely to be recalled when the passage is recalled.

Memory disorders

There exist certain disorders of explicit memory. The first of these is the amnestic syndrome, which is characterised by both an inability to learn new material (anterograde amnesia) and impaired recall of previously learned material (retrograde amnesia), with attendant lack of insight and confabulation. Implicit memory remains unaffected in such patients. There is little or no impairment in the function of STM.

In patients with dementia, the memory impairment is more diffuse and global, with recall and retention of events, regardless of recency, being progressively affected. STM – affected.

Finally, more specific memory loss may occur in psychogenic fugue where memory is generally unaffected except for specific items with personal meaning. This is commonly precipitated by some severe psychological or social stress.

Summary

- The most important model of memory to be aware of, and the most important distinction, is the two-stage (short-term memory/long-term memory) model proposed by Atkinson and Shiffrin. Information is suggested to be processed initially in a short-term store, being eventually consolidated into a long-term store. The use of short-term memory in psychology is quite different to the usage in psychiatry, referring to storage of only a few seconds duration. Short-term memory is also distinct from long-term memory in its capacity: only 7 ($\pm$ 2) items or units of information can be stored in short-term memory, while the capacity of long-term memory is theoretically limitless. Short-term memory capacity can be increased by chunking (i.e. grouping items of information into larger, single units).

- Short-term memory may also be referred to as 'primary' or 'working' memory. Baddeley's working memory model is the second model of memory to be aware of. This consists of a Central Executive overseeing the functioning of several modality specific information processing systems. The relationship between working memory and models of attention and information processing is a close one. This model does not alter the conception of long-term memory suggested by two-stage models of memory (i.e. Atkinson and Shiffrin).

- Distinguish between encoding, storage and retrieval – memory failure or inaccuracy may be due to failure at any of these three stages, and it is difficult to dissociate these experimentally and investigate them separately. Encoding refers to the initial processing of information in short-term memory, while retrieval refers to the process whereby information from long-term memory is returned to short-term memory. Storage obviously occurs in both short-term and long-term memory, but usually refers to long-term storage.

- Several types of memory have been distinguished, representing the organisational structure of long-term memory. Memories may be either explicit (able to be described by the individual) or implicit (evidenced by behaviour and not able to be described). Explicit, declarative memories include as subsets semantic memory for facts ('knowing that') and episodic memory for events. Implicit memories include procedural memory or memories for abilities and skills.

- Items in long-term memory are held in structured schemata or related groups, so that one item will bring to mind other, related items. These schemata are built up by a process of learning and association, and are therefore individual, while also being subject to cultural and social forces. Schemata exist for all types of memory, including procedural memories (in which case they are often referred to as 'scripts' for behaviour).

- Specific memory deficits exist in the amnestic syndrome, dementia and psychogenic fugue. Depressed subjects also show spontaneous recall of proportionally more negative, self-congruent material when compared with controls. This is a central feature of Beck's cognitive model of depression and is related to information processing biases in anxious subjects.

THOUGHT

Thought and language

The relationship between thought and language is a very close one, and while language is arguably not a uniquely human ability, it is fair to say that, at the very least, in humans it is most developed. While thought is evident in several forms (for example, imagery), the majority of human thinking is propositional. That is, thoughts are verbalised internally as a succession of sentences or monologues (or dialogues). The majority of research into thought, then, has focused on propositional thought. It is the communication of thought that is a function of language, and it should therefore not be surprising that the two interact so closely.

Concept, prototypes and cores

A *concept* may be described as a mental representation of a class of objects and is another example of the brain's ability to reduce information processing load. By treating all members of a class as broadly similar, the need for analysis of different situations is reduced, on the assumption that the members of that class will all behave in broadly similar ways in a given situation. A second function of concepts is to allow prediction, so that if an object is regarded as belonging to certain group certain characteristics that are not immediately obvious may be expected, given that those characteristics have been experienced in relation to other members of the group. The process whereby an object is assigned to a group is known as categorisation. Concepts may include physical objects, such as 'animal' or, more specifically, 'birds', or may be of more abstract ideas, such as 'democracy'.

For any given concept there will exist a prototype (sometimes known as an exemplar), which represents the best example of the concept. This prototype will be quite well defined, and as such will include properties that are not appropriate to the concept as a whole. For example, the prototype of 'bird' for a certain individual may be 'sparrow', although this is clearly incongruent with certain birds, such as penguins, since it includes the ability to fly. Therefore, prototypes are not necessarily logical or even strictly accurate examples of a member of a concept but represent the *popular* and best-recognised example. Prototypes can be accessed quite easily and are usually the words that come to mind when asked to think of specific concepts.

While *prototypes* are highly salient examples of a given concept, the properties are not necessary conditions for concept membership. This role is accomplished by the core properties of a concept, which represent the necessary and sufficient properties for an object to be included in a concept. The core of the concept 'widow', for example, might include properties such as female, husband deceased, and so on. Clearly, some concepts have more clear-cut cores than others, with 'widow' being an example of a well-defined concept with a limited number of unambiguous properties serving to completely define the concept.

Concepts and related features such as prototypes and cores serve an important function in determining thought and interpretation of language. For example, if told to think of a bird, one is far more likely to think of a sparrow than a penguin. Similarly, if asked whether a sparrow is a bird, the response of a subject is quicker than if asked whether a penguin is a bird. Adults notoriously misclassify whales and dolphins as fish, as they are examples that are very close, at least superficially, to the prototype of 'fish'. This goes some way to illustrating the distinction between the logical nature of a concept's core and the more subjective nature of a concept's prototype.

Deductive and inductive reasoning

A *deductive* argument is one where the conclusion *must* be true if the premises that lead to it are true. A simple example of a deductive argument might be:

A is greater than B; B is greater than C. Therefore, A is greater than C.

Adults are very good at determining the validity of simple deductive arguments, with this ability falling off as the number of premises (i.e. the difficulty of the argument) increases.

Inductive reasoning applies to arguments that may be strong but lack the logical rigour of deductive arguments. In this case, the argument is described as inductively strong (as opposed to weak), which simply allocates a very low probability to the possibility of the argument being false. Therefore, inductive reasoning is probabilistic. An example of an inductive argument might be:

A is usually greater than B; B is always greater than C. Therefore, A is greater than C.

When the premises of an argument are made explicit and the subject has time to reach a conclusion, deductive and inductive reasoning appear to be features of human thinking. However, this breaks down to an extent when everyday reasoning is considered; that is, although adult humans are clearly capable of reasoning deductively and inductively with a high degree of competence, these are not necessarily the forms of reasoning spontaneously adopted when confronted with a novel problem requiring a solution.

Problem-solving, algorithms and heuristics

When problem-solving in more realistic situations, individuals sometimes take short-cuts to arrive at conclusions, and these may violate the rules of deductive and inductive reasoning. This represents another example of reducing cognitive workload, and in general is advantageous as it allows (usually) accurate conclusions to be arrived at more quickly, although in specific instances the techniques employed may allow inaccurate conclusions to be arrived at. In general, two types of problem-solving techniques are employed: algorithmic techniques and heuristic techniques.

An *algorithm* represents a set of rules that, if applied stepwise, will always guarantee the solution of a problem. While a successful solution to the problem is guaranteed, the application may be inappropriate, for example if the time taken to complete the algorithm is too long. The best chess move from a given position may be computed algorithmically, but this is not an algorithm that a human could practically apply (although chess computers do so), since it requires calculating all possible moves from the current position, followed by all possible moves from the subsequent position, and so on for a number of specified iterations, with the chosen end state being evaluated. One should note that this highlights important differences in computer intelligence (as it currently stands) and human intelligence. In these cases heuristics, where problem-solving is directed but success is not guaranteed, would be more appropriate (for humans).

A *heuristic* represents a method for solving problems that rests on reducing the number of possibilities by initially discarding the most improbable and gradually focusing on the most likely. Taking the example of the chess game given above, a large number of moves, to the experienced player certainly, would be discarded immediately as inappropriate. This technique is best conceptualised as a 'rule of thumb' method, so that an adopted heuristic allows for an initial solution to be tested quite rapidly and then accepted or discarded.

The existence of prototypes (see above), however, can lead to errors in heuristics judgements. For example, if presented with the following statements and asked to judge the probabilities of each being correct:

'John is 25 years old and very popular. He is active and athletic, and studied computing at college'.

- John works for a computing consultancy.
- John works for a computing consultancy and plays football regularly.

Subjects are likely to rate the second option as more likely, even though this cannot be the case given that the second option requires two things to be true, while the first only requires one thing to be true. Presumably, the prototype generated by the second statement is closer to the description of John than the prototype generated by the first statement.

Therefore, while heuristic arguments (which depend on cognitive shortcuts such as prototypes) tend to produce useful solutions, their shortcomings become apparent in certain, usually experimental, instances. Nevertheless, in realistic situations such heuristics are a powerful problem-solving tool, often allowing humans to outperform computers using algorithms to solve an identical problem.

Summary

- Given the quantity of complexity of information that is continually being processed and stored, a high degree of organisation is essential. Related items of knowledge and classes of objects are represented by a concept that encapsulates the central features of the object class. Concepts may vary in degree of specificity and abstraction. A prototype exists as the best example of a concept, although it may contain features that are not universal to all members of the concept, and may be neither necessary nor sufficient. Those features of a concept that are necessary and sufficient for inclusion in the concept represent the core properties of the concept. A well-defined concept is one where the core properties may be readily listed.

- Two types of reasoning should be distinguished: a *deductive argument* is one where, if the premises are true the conclusion, logically, must be true (e.g. if A > B and if B > C, then A > C); an *inductive argument* is one where the conclusion does not follow necessarily from the premises if these are true, but instead is merely likely, so that a strong inductive argument is one where the probability of the conclusion being false is very low.

- Everyday problem-solving lacks the rigour of the two types of reasoning described. In this case, it is more useful to speak of algorithms and heuristics. An *algorithm* is a step of processes or operations that guarantees a successful solution to a specific problem (e.g. the best chess move by computing ALL possible moves). A *heuristic*, which characterises the majority of human problem-solving, is a cruder method for solving problems that does not guarantee success, but makes it likely in a far shorter period than a corresponding algorithm. Given the example of choosing a chess move, a human player would use heuristic thinking (immediately discarding a very large number of permissible but obviously valueless moves), while a computer would use an algorithmic process.

PERSONALITY

Nomothetic approaches

Any nomothetic (or nomological) theory is one that deals with abstract generalisations and universal concepts. Applied to personality theories, this incorporates theories that attempt to find patterns of behaviour across individuals that allow the personalities of all individuals to be classified according to a single system. Examples include trait and type theories.

Radiographic approaches

Radiographic (or idiographic) theories contrast with nomothetic theories in that they focus on the specific aspects of a given individual, on the assumption that the development of personality is too fluid to allow different individuals to be classified as the same along a certain dimension. Examples include psychoanalytic theories, personal construct theory and humanistic theories. These have the common feature of being difficult to refute or validate experimentally.

Trait and type approaches

Trait theories of personality assume that personality can be characterised by a small number of behavioural and cognitive dimensions. Statistical techniques, specifically factor analysis, are used to cluster descriptors, adjectives, or answers to questions, with these clusters corresponding to personality dimensions or traits. An example of a personality trait is the extraversion–introversion dimension, where individuals are classified according to their position along this dimension (determined usually by questionnaire). In the Eysenck Personality Questionnaire, for example, which includes an extraversion dimension, statements describing oneself or one's behaviour requiring a 'yes' or 'no' answer are marked to give a score where a higher score corresponds to higher levels of extraversion. Such questionnaires generally show good test-retest reliability, with scores measured at two different times typically correlating by 0.85, as long as the intervening period is not too great (i.e. not several years).

Type theories represent the oldest form of personality theory, with Hippocrates's description of four fundamental temperaments (sanguine, choleric, melancholy and phlegmatic) being an example. Essentially, this approach pigeonholes individuals on the basis of the pattern of personality characteristics that they demonstrate. An example is the Type A individual, who is characterised as highly driven, competitive and time-oriented. Personality type (such as the Type A personality) can be assessed either by means of a self-report questionnaire or an assessment checklist that is completed by an observer. The limitation of types theories is that they only allow for limited individual variation within the type, at least in terms of the defining characteristics of the type, so that they offer poorer sensitivity to differences between individuals than trait theories.

It is important to realise that these two approaches are by no means exclusive; indeed, the two may be regarded as highly complementary, with type theories attempting to discern commonalities across individuals and trait theories attempting to achieve greater discrimination between individuals. Type theories may be regarded as at the top of a hierarchy, with trait theories representing a further analysis, at one level below in the hierarchy, followed by general responses and then responses specific to a given situation.

The use of factor analysis in the construction of such models of personality creates problems of interpretation, as well as the reliance on this technique of adequate initial data. Such models fail to take into account the demands of the situation (although this is not what they aim to do) and often give poor discriminatory power, especially if the number of dimensions is few.

Personal construct theory

Personal construct theory is typified by an emphasis on the self-image individuals have of themselves, in particular by allowing the individual to construct the dimensions along which the personality characteristics are to be mapped (in contrast to the dimensions which the experimenter offers to the subject in trait approaches). Typical theories of personality, in particular trait and type theories, are rejected by personal construct theory on the grounds that they do not allow the individual to assess personality on one's own terms and instead impose an external frame of reference.

The test used in personal construct theory is the repertory grid (see below) which allows the central themes which characterise the individual to be explored using the individual's own terms. The test is not restricted to individuals and may also be used in the consideration of events, and is used in both research and counselling. Possible problems with this approach include the questionable reliability of this method: a grid constructed at time 1 may not yield similar results to one constructed at time 2. Also, the criticism that trait approaches do not allow for the expression of one's individual sense of personality, while valid, overlooks the fact the external judgement of personality by an external observer can be of greater importance in certain situations.

Psychoanalytic approaches

Psychoanalytic theories of personality (also known as psychodynamic theories) stem from the work of Freud and Jung, and share the common element that personality is seen as a developmental process driven by underlying motivational factors. Freud in particular emphasised that all human behaviour, thought and emotion is caused mostly by unconscious drives and motivations. Personality, in Freudian theory, consists of three interacting components:

- The Id represents the primitive personality from which other aspects of personality develop and constitutes the basic biological drives, such as eating and sexual behaviour.
- The Ego represents the aspect of the personality which oversees the others and judges which actions should be performed and which should not.
- The Superego, finally, is the moral aspect of the personality which determines whether an action is right or wrong.

These elements are suggested to develop through five stages of psychosexual development, through which nearly all children pass in the following order:

- *Oral*, for approximately the first 18 months of life, where activities concerning the mouth, lips, etc. provide satisfaction and interest.
- *Anal*, from approximately 18 to 36 months, at the stage when toilet training occurs and control over this activity offers an expression of independence.
- *Phallic*, from approximately 3 to 6 years, where the main source of satisfaction arises from the genitals.
- *Latency*, following the phallic stage and up to puberty, where sexual feelings are minimal and boys and girls tend to socialise and play separately.
- *Genital*, from puberty onwards, when once again the genitals are the main source of satisfaction, with the emphasis now on pleasure with another rather than alone.

Psychoanalytic theories suffer from difficulty in testing the predictions that arise from them, not least because of the difficulty in accurately assessing the childhood experiences that the theory would predict would have an impact on adult personality. Where such testing is possible there is often only negative evidence for the theory.

Humanistic approaches

The humanistic approach, associated primarily with Carl Rogers (1902–1987) and Abraham Maslow (1908–1970), rests on four principles:

- The individual and the individual's subjective experience are of prime interest, and behavioural and cognitive approaches do not do justice to the richness of individual differences.
- Creativity and choice represent the ideals of personality (as opposed to the conflicts of psychoanalytic theories).
- The problem should guide research, rather than the research method. That is, psychology should not be regarded as a value-free science and should investigate problems of real importance.
- Individuals are essentially good (unlike in psychoanalytic theories where individuals are essentially bad or aggressive).

Personality theories based on this approach emphasise the role of the self-concept, representing the individual's conception of the values and ideas characterising oneself, and value introspection as a means of understanding that which motivates human behaviour. This self-concept, in turn, influences perception of the world and the individual's own behaviour within it. One individual with a concept of him/herself as confident will act in a very different way to another individual who regards him/herself as shy and diffident.

Rogers suggested that the individual strives for congruence between the self-concept and the ideal self. Acting in a way incongruent with the ideal self results in anxiety that must be resolved, for example by denial. The approach of Maslow emphasised the need for self-actualisation (see Motivation, p. 40), which is the pinnacle of one's potential and can be achieved only after a more basic hierarchy of needs are met (see Motivation, p. 40).

Interactionist approaches

Interactionist approaches, unlike the highly focused theories described above, accept certain features from several theories. Central to these approaches is the assumption that behaviour results from an interaction between aspects of the individual and the specifics of the situation. As such, it is unwise to search for 'personality' as a distinct entity, given that whatever constitutes personality is likely to depend to a significant extent on interaction with the environment. In this sense, personality can only be inferred from consistency of behaviours, but is unlikely to ever provide any great predictive or explanatory power.

- *Reactive interaction* is the extent to which we interact with subjective interpretations of a given situation.
- *Evocative interaction* represents the extent to which the behaviour of an individual elicits behaviours from others.
- *Proactive interaction* accounts for the degree to which situations congruent with consistent behaviours/personality are sought out by the individual.

Inventories, rating scales, grids and Q-sort

In personality theory, an inventory is a battery of questions that assesses personality following the trait or type approach. Typically, a large number of questions are administered to a large group of individuals, and the responses then clustered by the statistical technique of factor analysis. Redundant items are removed and the clusters named as specific dimensions (e.g. extraversion–introversion).

Shortcomings of this approach include the question of how the initial battery of questions is selected, and the subjectivity involved in naming the clusters as dimensions. Note that the factor is not equivalent to the trait, but instead the trait is inferred from the factor. In other words, the factor is a behavioural reflection of the underlying trait, which may be a biological (and, perhaps, partly heritable) difference or simply consistency in behaviour, depending on the theoretical stance adopted.

An alternative means of trait measurement allows for more degrees of freedom in answering specific items. Rather than the common 'yes'/'no' options presented with items on many tests, rating scales allow, for example, for the frequency of specific behaviours to be rated. In the case of self-related statements, the subject may be asked to what extent he agrees or disagrees with each statement, for example on a 5-point scale.

The *repertory grid*, which is the tool used in personal construct theory, most commonly compares several close friends, lovers, family and so on along dimensions chosen by the subject. Three individuals are chosen where two share a personality characteristic and the third contrasts with this. For example, 'myself' and 'best friend' may be described as extraverted, while 'neighbour' may be described as introverted. This process continues for each row that exists in the resulting matrix.

The *Q-sort technique*, used by humanistic psychologists, also gives control over the personality assessment process to the subject. In this case, several cards, each containing a personality descriptor, are given to the subject whose task is to sort the cards into piles containing phrases that most describe and least describe an individual, with the remaining cards being placed in intermediate piles. Two Q-sorts can be compared by calculating correlations between scores on both sorts (allocated on the basis of which pile an item is in).

If the two Q-sorts an individual is asked to construct are 'ideal self' and 'actual self', the correlation between the two is the self-ideal discrepancy. A low or negative correlation would be expected to be related to feelings of low self-esteem, according to Rogers. This has also been used to assess the ongoing efficacy of Rogerian client-centred therapy.

Summary

- There are several approaches to the study of personality: the nomothetic deals with universal patterns of behaviour that can be used to described all individuals. Within this approach there are trait and type theories, which are themselves complementary. *Trait theories* propose a small number of independent personality dimensions along which any given individual can vary. The pattern of variation along these dimensions is supposed to present a comprehensive description of an individual's personality. *Type theories* suggest that a small number of personality types exist, encompassing all variation in human personality. Trait and type theories are complementary in that a certain pattern of trait characteristics may be suggested to correspond with a certain personality type. An alternative approach to personality theory is the *radiographic*, where each individual is analysed separately and no generalisations are made. Psychoanalytic, personal construct and humanistic theories serve as examples of this kind of approach.
- Personal construct theory emphasises an individual's self-appraisal in studying personality, allowing the individual to construct the dimensions to be used to assess personality. The *repertory grid* is the principal tool used in the construction of these dimensions.
- One should be aware of the basic principles of psychoanalytic, humanistic and interactionist theories of personality. All of these share the common characteristic of being difficult to prove or refute. *Psychoanalytic theories* suggest a central role for unconscious drives and desires as the motive force behind behaviour and, therefore, personality. *Humanistic theories* contrast with psychoanalytic theories in that they suggest humans to be essentially good (as opposed to aggressive and driven by primal instincts). *Interactionist approaches* represent a compromise whereby several theories are drawn on in order to explain the behaviour of an individual in any given situation (rather than searching for personality *per se*).
- Assessment of personality will depend on the approach being taken, with questionnaires being favoured by trait and type theories and more complex tools, such as the repertory grid or Q-sort, being favoured by radiographic approaches.

MOTIVATION

Needs and drives

A need–drive model is one that proposes that specific physiological needs (e.g. water) are produced when what is needed is lacking. These needs result in drives, and it is these that motivate behaviour, being directed towards the resolution of the need. Physiological models suggest a role for the hypothalamus in mediating this relationship (see below), particularly in the case of feeding. It has also been suggested that these basic needs underlie all motivational behaviour, and that secondary reinforcers (such as money) are effective reinforcers which motivate behaviour in the same ways as basic drives because, ultimately, they also allow a basic need to be resolved (see below).

Extrinsic theories

If the motivation for an action (i.e. the reward for behaviour or punishment for non-behaviour that may result) is external, the behaviour is said to be *extrinsically motivated*. An athlete will train for success in competition (or through fear of failure), with satisfaction at personal fitness and health interests being only secondary.

Physiological needs which may be satisfied by external objects such as food or water result in primary drives (i.e. those required to survive and innate). Secondary drives result when primary drives become associated (through conditioning processes) with other objects. For example, money is sought not because it satisfies any primary needs but because of what it is associated with, and because it allows primary needs to be resolved indirectly (e.g. by allowing one to buy food). As such, there will be substantial individual differences in secondary drives as a result of developmental learning processes.

Homeostasis

Broadly, homeostasis is used to refer to a process whereby change in a system results in further processes that restore the system to the initial state; a mechanical analogue would be a thermostat.

In the case of theories of motivation, homeostasis refers to the process whereby basic needs are self-regulating, so that thirst is the consequence of insufficient water being ingested, which can then be satisfied by drinking water, and homeostasis is restored. Drinking serves as a good example of a homeostatic mechanism as it is maintained and positively reinforced by factors such as the taste of water, which becomes more pleasant as thirst increases.

Hypothalamic systems and satiety

There is substantial evidence that the control mechanism of homeostasis, particularly in the case of feeding, resides in the hypothalamus. Animal studies suggest that damage to certain areas of the hypothalamus (ventral and medial hypothalamus) results in insatiable appetite and gross overeating. Damage to other areas of the hypothalamus (lateral hypothalamus) results in the converse condition where the animal will ignore food and display no apparent appetite.

While the hypothalamus is clearly important in the regulation of eating, it is not the sole area of importance. This is evidenced by the gradual restoration of appetite of animals with hypothalamic lesions. The system is clearly an interactive one and hypothalamic lesions, rather than simply removing or exacerbating appetite, rather serve to reset parameters in the homeostasis of hunger.

Intrinsic theories

Any behaviour that is intrinsically motivated is dependent on internal factors, in particular subjective feelings of success, satisfaction, and so on. The behaviour is satisfying or rewarding in itself, rather than achieving some external goal that provides satisfaction. Examples include psychosocial motivators such as need for achievement (see below), and related concepts such as needs for affiliation (social contact) and intimacy (closeness). There are substantial individual differences in the absolute and relative importance of these intrinsic motivators. Attachment behaviour in early life may be regarded as another example of an apparently intrinsic primary drive.

Curiosity

The tendency to seek novel stimuli is commonly regarded as innate, although inferring curiosity in animal studies may be problematic. In the context of motivation, this represents a shortcoming of purely extrinsic theories of motivation, since curiosity is satisfied internally by the activity that it elicits. While it may be argued in some instances that secondary drives result from conditioning processes and primary drives, this does not appear to hold in the case of curiosity, which appears to be a primary drive but not one motivated by a physiological need. Similar arguments are relevant to understanding psychosocial drives such as need for affiliation or attachment theory. The latter is particularly interesting when one considers evidence from animal studies that suggests that an infant animal will seek an attachment figure that offers comfort rather than a figure that offers food (see below).

Optimal levels of arousal

The Yerkes–Dodson law suggests that performance level follows a curvilinear relationship (as an inverted U) with arousal (defined broadly to include motivation, anxiety, etc.), so that optimal performance exists at a moderate level of arousal, with poorer performance being associated with excessively low or excessively high arousal. Although this law is empirically well supported, it should be noted that it is descriptive, rather than explanatory.

Different individuals are suggested, by this theory, to have different levels of optimal arousal, which in turn determine behaviour. Sensation-seeking individuals, with a high optimal level of arousal, will therefore seek out behaviours to satisfy this, such as parachute jumping. Eysenck has incorporated this into a model of personality (extraversion–introversion dimension). Evidence in support of this comes from, among other sources, radar operators who showed great variance in efficiency in studies carried out during the Second World War. Those individuals who were highly introverted sustained attention for longer periods presumably, by this theory, because less stimulation was required to sustain interest, while extraverted individuals sought stimulation elsewhere. Need for achievement has also been suggested as a personality dimension of relevance to motivation and performance (see below).

Limitations to these approaches

There are certain shortcomings to the above approaches, such as the need to include behaviours which do not fulfil any physiological needs (curiosity, attachment behaviour) as primary drives. In the case of attachment behaviours in animals, rhesus monkeys deprived of their mother will seek comfort from a fur model that does not provide food rather than a wire model that does provide food, although they will seek the wire model when hungry or thirsty to satisfy these needs, after which they will return to the fur model. This suggests, at the very least, that the definition of what constitutes a drive must be broad and flexible so as to incorporate such psychosocial and emotional drives.

Also, drive reduction is not a necessary condition for behaviour to be learned – vicarious learning (modelling), for example, is possible.

There are three areas that must be incorporated in any complete understanding of motivation:

- Physiological needs may be explained with reference to primary drives (but see above considerations).
- The integration of drive theory and learning theory allows for an understanding of secondary drives and more complex behaviour.
- Finally, psychosocial explanations of highly complex behaviours are required, such as social learning theory, in particular for understanding uniquely human behaviour.

Cognitive consistency

Cognitive dissonance is the result of two incompatible beliefs being held, or a belief held which is inconsistent with current behaviour. Reduction of this dissonance may be regarded as a drive motivating behaviour, and cognitive dissonance theory holds that there exists a basic (psychosocial) need in humans for consistency in thinking, reasoning and behaviour. Given that cognitive consistency (the opposite of dissonance) is sought, when dissonance exists (for example, as a result of engaging in a behaviour that is contrary to a firmly held attitude) the individual must either reappraise the relevant beliefs/cognitions or change behaviour. It is in this sense that cognitive consistency may be regarded as a need, consequently motivating behaviour.

Need for achievement

Another cognitive model of motivation is the 'need for achievement' (or nAch), which is suggested to represent a personality trait that incorporates a desire to master difficult tasks and overcome obstacles. This is related to an individual's concept of a self-ideal, incorporating personal standards that represent success or achievement. Allied to this is the drive to work towards this ideal, such that the ideal may be regarded as a need, with discrepancy from this ideal resulting in drive. This is assessed by means of the Thematic Apperception Test, which require participants to relate a story to each of a series of pictures. A consistent theme of achievement indicates a high nAch.

It is potentially restrictive to consider achievement as the only complex human need: several other psychosocial needs also exist, such as group membership, self-esteem and so on, some of which have been described above.

Maslow's hierarchy of needs

The suggestion of this conception of motivation is that there exists a pyramid of needs, with those lower in the hierarchy being more closely related to innate, physiological needs. These, then, must be satisfied before it is possible to attempt satisfaction of higher order needs. The highest level of need, self-actualisation, was investigated by Maslow by asking participants to report their 'peak experiences', affective states of extreme euphoria that occur only rarely and on occasions that are subjectively associated with a sensation of being absolutely satisfied and content.

- Self-actualisation   –   achievement, etc.
- Aesthetic   –   symmetry, order.
- Cognitive   –   knowledge, understanding.
- Self-esteem   –   social acceptance, recognition.
- Belonging/social   –   group membership, affiliation.
- Safety   –   security, absence of danger.
- Physical/physiological –   hunger, thirst, sex.

As with other humanistic approaches, this model suffers from a heavy reliance on subjective experience, and a lack of empirically testable predictions arising from it. Nevertheless, by highlighting the role of important psychosocial drives it represents an important part of our understanding of human motivation.

Summary

- Theories of motivation may be extrinsic or intrinsic. *Extrinsic theories* suggest that the motivation for a given behaviour is external to the organism (e.g. reward or punishment). *Intrinsic theories* suggest a role for internal factors such as hunger, curiosity, etc.
- Certain basic needs, such as hunger and thirst, are self-regulating: *homeostasis* refers to this process of self-regulation, whereby change in a system results in further, compensatory change. Research on animal subjects suggests that the control of this process resides in the hypothalamus, apparently serving to set the parameters within which fluctuation occurs.
- There are certain shortcomings to simple models of motivation. Most importantly, certain behaviours appear to be primary drives without fulfilling any physiological need. Examples include curiosity and attachment behaviour. In humans, *cognitive consistency* and the *need for achievement* (nAch) also appear to be important determinants of behaviour. While certain behaviours may be learned by the association of these with primary drive reduction, it seems that complex social

behaviours also serve to reduce primary drives, so that emotional proximity, for example, may represent a primary drive which is reduced by attachment behaviour.

- The complex pattern of primary and secondary drives may be clarified to some extent by Maslow's hierarchy of needs, which suggest that basic drives must be satisfied initially before it becomes possible to divert attention to higher order needs, such as social acceptance, group membership, and so on.

EMOTION

Components of emotional response

Defining emotion is not straightforward, but it is reasonable to suggest that any emotional response may be regarded as consisting of four components:

- Subjective feeling
- Physiological response
- Behavioural response (or *readiness* to behave)
- Cognitive response

It is the pattern of interaction between these components that constitutes an emotion or emotional response. An important issue is the extent to which these components influence each other; for example, is one more likely to become angry if in a state of high autonomic arousal, for example athletes in competition?

It should be noted that emotions are generally stimulated externally, are acute and intense, and can therefore be distinguished from moods, which tend to be self-perpetuating, less intense and persist for longer periods. They are also functional, at least in appropriate contexts, so that fear, for example, is accompanied by changes (physiological, behavioural, etc.) that allow a response to meet the threat posed by the source of the fear (the 'fight or flight' syndrome).

James–Lange theory

Ext. events → Beh./Phys. changes → Emot.

Emotion, by this theory, is construed as resulting directly from behavioural or physiological changes that occur in response to external events, which are perceived by the subject so that the emotion is the subjective feeling of that change. While there are some physiological correlates of emotion (e.g. adrenaline and fear, noradrenaline and anger, cortisol and anxiety) these tend to be the exception rather than the rule.

Criticisms include the generality of some physiological responses across a range of emotions, which can sometimes include contradictory ones (e.g. fear and extreme happiness both elicit elevated pulse). External manipulation of physiological correlates of emotion, for example the injection of adrenaline, does not elicit the corresponding emotion (although an emotion can be cued in such circumstances by telling the participant that the injection which is to follow can stimulate a given emotion). Finally, emotional changes take place far more quickly than physiological responses.

Cannon–Bard theory

This is also known as the 'thalamic theory of emotion', since it suggests that emotion is controlled by the thalamus by stimulating the cortex, with the hypothalamus controlling any attendant behaviour. The behavioural and physiological changes resulting from specific emotions are, therefore, secondary to the emotion.

This may be criticised on the basis that although the physiological correlates of emotion may be more complex than suggested by the James–Lange theory, they are nevertheless far from secondary (see below, Differentiation).

Cognitive appraisal

Any given situation or stimulus is suggested by this theory to evoke a physiological response, accompanied by a cognitive appraisal of the physiological response and the situation as threatening, good, etc. It should be noted that the same physiological response can, therefore, elicit different emotions as a function of the attendant cognitive appraisal.

Differentiation

Within any given culture individuals are highly skilled at differentiating emotions in others on the basis of observed behaviour, in particular facial expression. Moreover, many of these emotions show corresponding physiological changes that, although more complex than suggested by the James–Lange theory, are nevertheless distinctive. Heart rate, for example, while increasing for both negative and positive emotions, appears to increase significantly more for negative emotions (e.g. fear) than positive emotions (e.g. happiness). Finally, certain basic emotions appear to be universal across cultures and show similarly universal patterns of physiological change (see below).

Perhaps more important than physiological change in the differentiation of emotions is the role of *cognitive appraisal* (see above). For example, the fear associated with a parachute jump would be far greater for a novice than for an experienced individual. The role of cognition and cognitive appraisal is also important in theories of panic and other emotional disorders.

Primary emotions

There is substantial evidence, especially from cross-cultural studies, that there are a limited number of basic emotions that are universal. Other more complex forms of emotional expression are culturally learned, and therefore difficult to interpret by other cultures. Darwin argued that each emotion is discrete and is associated with a characteristic and unique behavioural expression. Although there is debate over the exact number of primary, universal emotions (with corresponding primary and universal expressions), the following is a representative list:

- Sadness
- Joy
- Fear
- Anger
- Disgust
- Anticipation
- Surprise
- Trust

Emotion and performance

Related to any discussion of basic emotions is the question of what function these emotions serve, and their value to the individual who experiences the emotion. From an evolutionary perspective emotions may be seen as prompting behaviour that is appropriate in a given situation and preparing the organism accordingly. Fear, for example, elicits a very strong sympathetic reaction, which in turn prepares the organism to react to the threatening stimulus, either by confronting it or retreating (fight-or-flight). Other emotional responses, in particular negative ones such as sadness, may be associated with a parasympathetic response.

Summary

- Two early theories of emotion are important: the *James–Lange theory* suggested that emotion is the result of physiological or behavioural change, which is associated with the subjective feelings of a corresponding emotion; the *Cannon–Bard theory* suggested that emotion is distinct from the physiological and behavioural changes associated with it, being the result of activity in the thalamus and cortex. The former theory ascribes to central a role for the physiological and behavioural correlates of emotion, while the latter regards these as too peripheral.

- There is substantial evidence for the existence of a limited number (the exact number is debatable) of primary emotions that are universal across cultures. These include, in most studies, emotions such as fear, anger, joy, etc.

- Emotions are complex and consist of related, interacting components: the subjective feeling, while being the most apparent feature of emotions, is the most difficult to investigate. More amenable to investigation are the physiological, behavioural and cognitive components. Any emotional response will include all of these features; anxiety, for example, may be characterised by specific physiological changes (e.g. cortisol secretion) as well as cognitive changes (e.g. preferential attention towards threatening material).

STRESS

Physiological aspects

Stress may be defined initially as any condition where perceived demand outstrips perceived resources. It should be noted that the appraisal of the situation by the organism is therefore important. This fact is central to understanding stress, given that there is enormous individual difference in the quality and quantity of stress response to any given environmental change or stimulus.

Any stressor (i.e. object that causes stress) elicits a general physiological reaction – the General Adaptation Syndrome (GAD), or fight–flight response. The sympathetic and adrenal-cortical systems act to prepare the organism for responding to an acute physical threat, so that this general response has a clear evolutionary purpose.

The response may not always be appropriate, however, if the stressor is chronic or non-physical in nature, in which case the sustained elevated arousal resulting from this response may ultimately have negative effects on health. While the initial reaction may be called the alarm reaction (the first stage of the GAD), this cannot be sustained indefinitely and the organism will eventually move to the second stage (resistance) where arousal is lowered but remains higher than normal. Finally, if the stressor remains present, the third stage, exhaustion, results. It is at this stage that illness is suggested by the GAD model to be more likely in those suffering from chronic stress.

Psychological aspects

While the physiological reaction to a stressor is general, the range of psychological reactions to the same stressor is far broader and varies widely across individuals and situations. Common reactions to stressor include:

- Anxiety
- Aggression
- Depression

The onset of major depression is often preceded by a stressful life event, while post-traumatic stress disorder is now a widely accepted diagnostic category as a result of evidence from disaster victims and individuals in war zones (military and civilian) where a particularly severe stressor results in chronic anxiety, sleep disturbances, and so on.

Equally, however, some individuals thrive on stress and challenge (see below: Coping mechanisms, Locus of control). Environmental challenges that one individual might find distressing may be found by another as rewarding and stimulating. It is for this reason that care must be taken in the use of the word and concept 'stress', given that there is an important difference between the degree of challenge and the impact of this on a given individual. The interactive nature of stress means that even the degree of environmental challenge cannot be measured objectively, as it will be interpreted differently by varying individuals and therefore *be* different to those individuals.

Situational factors

Early research into stress focused on the role of major stressors and life events. The Social Readjustment Rating Scale contains several items scored for stressfulness, where subjects are required to mark items that have occurred to them in the last year. The stressfulness score can then be calculated to assess the level of stress for each individual. An obvious weakness (and there are several) of the SRRS is that it does not account for the subjective appraisal of the stressor by the individual. As mentioned earlier, what is threatening for one individual may be challenging and stimulating for another, so that a specific event will affect different individuals in different ways. Moreover, reactions to major life events will depend also on factors such as social support, so that divorce is likely to be more distressing for an individual with little social support.

More recent theories of stress emphasise the role of 'daily hassles' rather than major life events. These hassles are usually chronic in nature and yet not severe enough in themselves to warrant concern from others, which in part accounts for their impact in that they do not elicit the support that can ameliorate the impact of a major life event. The association between physical health and stress is stronger if the measure of stress used is a daily hassles score rather than a life events score. Examples of daily hassles include regularly being delayed in traffic, conflict at work or home and continual time urgency.

One extension of this theory is the incorporation of 'daily uplifts' as being minor desirable events that improve mood for a short period. These have been shown to be (negatively) correlated with poor physical health, representing a protective factor.

Distinct from these normal stressors are those that may be regarded as in some sense catastrophic and traumatic. Examples of these include major accidents (road, air, etc.), terrorist bombings, and so on. The features of events that contribute to their stressfulness, such as unpredictability and negativity, are particularly strong in these cases, and the reaction of individuals correspondingly strong, with post-traumatic stress disorder being a common consequence of such stressors. Distress following such events may remain for over a year after the event.

Vulnerability and invulnerability

Individual differences in reactions to specific stressors are substantial, and this is reflected in the extent to which negative emotions or physical ill-health result from stressful events. Certainly there are individual differences in susceptibility to stress-related illnesses, both physical and mental.

Invulnerability (or hardiness) represents the extent to which the individual's personality and subjective appraisal of stressful events contributes to the resilience of the organism, acting as a protective factor. Perceiving threat, in particular change, as a challenge and having a subjective sense of control over oneself and one's future are major factors contributing to invulnerability.

Similarly, perceiving change as threatening and feeling unable to control events contributes to *vulnerability* and a susceptibility to stress-related illness. There is some evidence that these psychological mediators of the stress response have physiological correlates, for example 'invulnerable' individuals show less elevation of heart rate in a stressful situation than 'vulnerable' individuals.

Type A behaviour

Given these individual differences in appraisal of and reaction to stressors, there is substantial interest in the role of personality factors more generally in mediating stress reactions. Most common of these is the Type A personality or behaviour pattern, characterised by:

- Drive, often excessive
- Competitiveness
- Ambition
- Time urgency
- Emphasis on quantity rather than quality
- Distractibility
- Hostility

Of particular interest is the well-established relationship between type A behaviour and coronary heart disease, with type A behaviour representing a significant risk factor. Of current interest is the extent to which these behavioural and personality differences are related to physiological differences, in particular individual differences in sympathetic nervous system reactivity.

Coping mechanisms

A *coping response* is a behavioural or cognitive reaction to a stressor designed to counter the stressor and meet the perceived demands of the situation. For example, work demands may result in several hours of overtime to compensate. There are numerous definitions and distinctions used in the study of coping. Most usefully, these are:

- Problem-focused
- Emotion-focused

Problem-focused strategies include those which seek to change the stressor or its effect on the individual, for example by retreating or removing the stressor. *Emotion-focused strategies* seek to modify the reaction of the individual but do not change the stressor, examples being the use of drugs (especially alcohol) or distraction techniques. In other words, when presented with a stressful situation, the individual may change the actual situation itself (problem-focused) or his/her response to it (emotion-focused).

Locus of control

Generally, this is the perceived control an individual has over oneself and the environment. It is a dimensional concept, with the extremes being internal control and external control. Internal control is related to a sense of responsibility for one's own actions and a feeling of being in control over one's environment. Conversely, an external locus of control reflects a sense that events are determined by external factors and success (or failure) is beyond the control of the individual. It is important to note that this is not an objective assessment of control but a subjective one.

In relation to stress, internal control beliefs tend to be associated with positive responses to stressors, while external locus of control is related to poor adjustment and coping.

Learned helplessness and learned resourcefulness

In the original study of learned helplessness, two dogs were 'yoked' so that each received identical electric shocks, the only difference between the dogs being that one was able to turn off the shock (for itself and the other dog), while the other was not. Therefore, the intensity and duration of shock received by each dog was identical, but one had control over the situation and the other did not. When placed in a different situation where avoidance was this time possible for both dogs, the dog that previously had no control exhibited helplessness and passivity to the extent that avoidance from the shock was not attempted. This learned helplessness may be prevented from developing by introducing a few trials where both dogs have control, so that an apparently opposite condition of learned resourcefulness develops.

While this research was intended to provide an analogue for human depression, the implications are far broader. Importantly, helplessness learned in one situation generalises to others. The general apathy and depression following stressful events may be explicable in terms of a learned helplessness model, in particular the behaviour found in, for example, women in violent relationships.

Summary

- Stress should be understood in the context of two literatures: the *psychological* and the *physiological*. Obviously the two overlap, but the relationship between the two has sometimes been a strained one (!) The general adaptation syndrome (GAD), or fight-flight response, exists in animals and humans, while it is difficult to ascribe subjective emotional states such as anxiety to animals, at least in a quantitative way.
- The study of stress is further complicated by the lack of any simple main effects: the characteristics of the individual will interact with *environmental* and *situational* variables, resulting in stress (or the lack of it) in response to a potential stressor. These individually will include, for example, the behavioural response generally adapted by an individual when confronted with a potential stressor (e.g. Type A personality). Life events scales which allocate a value to particular events are limited in that they do not take into account the specific effect of that event on an individual, the context within which it occurs, and so on.
- *Coping behaviour* may be characterised in a number of ways: active/passive, emotion-focused/problem-focused, vigilant/avoidant, etc. It is also important to understand the extent to which individual differences in locus of control (extent to which the individual perceives the environment as controllable), self-efficacy (extent to which the individual feels able to exert control) and learned helplessness (generalised expectation of helplessness as a result of learning) mediate the response to potential stressors. Note the converse of learned helplessness (i.e. learned resourcefulness).

STATES AND LEVELS OF AWARENESS

Levels of consciousness

Consciousness is not a dichotomous, 'on-off' concept; instead, one must speak of levels of consciousness (cf. Freud's use of unconscious and pre-conscious). This is not always apparent, particularly in common use where consciousness implies awareness. More accurately, the level of consciousness may vary from complete lack of awareness (unconscious) to high sensitivity to external events (hyperconsciousness, or the hyperacusis found in manic patients).

Consciousness has two roles, related to concepts of attention and information processing:
- Monitoring information
- Controlling behaviour

Unconscious processing

Given the quantity of information present at any given time, only a small proportion can be consciously processed. The process of initial selection and rejection of information takes place before these items enter full consciousness, i.e. at a preconscious stage. There is substantial evidence that learning and other information processing takes place without the awareness of the individual. For example, there is some evidence that anaesthetised subjects retain some information processing functions – generally those which are more primitive and robust.

A distinction should be made between preconscious processing and subconscious processing: the preconscious stage is that immediately prior to the conscious and contains information which may be accessed consciously but is not currently being so accessed; the subconscious stage filters information which never reaches full consciousness but selects items for processing, so that one's name may be recognised in a conversation which was not being attended to.

These levels of pre- and subconsciousness are distinct from unconscious processing. Freud's initial use of 'the unconscious' emphasised its role in driving emotional responses. More currently, unconscious processing refers to all information, learned associations and so on which influence behaviour without being consciously accessible. For example, ball catching is a skill most individuals possess to a greater or lesser degree, but we are unaware of the projectile calculations required to perform such a feat, even though in some sense they must be performed.

Arousal, attention and alertness

Arousal, generally, refers to the level of activity, along a dimension, based on sensory sensitivity, autonomic activity, and so on. This may be altered pharmacologically or by external events, given that humans usually exist in a moderate state of arousal, with scope for both increases and decreases in this level.

Attention, unlike arousal, does not vary in quantity so much as in quality. Given the extent to which selectivity is necessary for efficient information processing different aspects of the environment will command more or less attentional resources as a function of the current needs of the organism. Therefore, a hungry organism will selectively attend to objects that may be edible, largely at a subconscious level so that such objects are preferentially passed into consciousness.

Alertness is best regarded as a conjunction of arousal and attention, so that a high level of alertness consists of increased arousal and increased attention, as well as a focusing of attentional resources towards relevant stimuli. An example might be a hunted organism where a very high state of arousal will exist as well as extreme sensitivity to a very narrow range of stimuli.

Sleep structure

Sleeping individuals also display levels of consciousness in that some appear to be sleeping far more deeply than others. Furthermore, this depth of sleep may vary within individuals over time. Sleep structure may be broken down as follows:

- Stage 1   –   early sleep, EEG less regular and reduced in amplitude.
- Stage 2   –   short regular patterns of 12–16 Hz (spindles).
- Stage 3   –   deep sleep, long wavelength rhythms 1–2 Hz, delta waves – common (20–30%).
- Stage 4   –   deep sleep, similar to stage 3, delta waves more common (50+%).
- REM   –   rapid eye movement, noticeable through eyelids, dreams common.

The four stages of sleep are classified as NREM (or non-REM) sleep to distinguish them from REM sleep. The deeper the sleep (i.e. later stages), the more difficult the subject is to wake. Subjects woken from NREM sleep report dreams in about 25% of cases, whereas dream report almost always occurs when a subject is woken from REM sleep.

Dreaming

Freudian theory suggests that dreams represent manifestations of suppressed desires, wishes, etc. What is known to the dreamer is the manifest content, while the aspects requiring interpretation are the latent content.

More current theories of dreaming hypothesise a cognitive restructuring function. This may either take the form of information being sorted and stored, with dreams reflecting on a small proportion of the overall restructuring that takes place. Alternatively, dreams have been suggested to be the by-product of a neural 'cleaning' process where extraneous material is removed (rather than simply restructured). The activity required for this to take place results in dreaming.

Parasomnias

Psychological stress and biological factors are thought to be responsible for disturbances during sleep such as terror, where the individual is difficult to wake and usually recalls little of the incident, and sleepwalking. These occur during NREM, short-wavelength sleep (i.e. stages 1 and 2). During REM sleep nightmares and anxiety attacks may occur, with recall of the incident being very vivid.

Narcolepsy is frequently associated with affective or personality disorders and is characterised by hypersomnolence, with onset being sudden and usually irresistible.

Biorhythms

A large number of biological systems display some degree of periodicity, and a general label for this phenomenon is biorhythms, an example being the menstrual cycle. Current interest is largely focused on the circadian rhythms, which are daily fluctuations in functions such as temperature, blood pressure, hormone release, and so on. Experiments where subjects are removed from natural day/night variation suggest that the natural period of these rhythms slightly longer than 25 hours, so that these rhythms are maintained without external reinforcement but are recalibrated daily in normal circumstances.

Sleep deprivation

Sleep deprivation results in disruption of cognitive and motor performance, becoming marked after just 12–24 hours of sleep deprivation. Interestingly, only a proportion of lost sleep (25–30%) is ultimately regained by those undergoing sleep deprivation, suggesting a distinction between core sleep, which is essential for normal functioning and the remaining extraneous hours which most adults sleep through (average 8 hours). This is supported by evidence that as little sleep as 5 hours may be tolerated if achieved gradually.

Hypnosis and suggestibility

Suggestibility as a general term refers to the extent to which an individual is responsive to the suggestions of others. In a more technical sense it is related to hypnosis, a term with unfortunate associations. It is now broadly accepted that a hypnotic state does exist, characterised by:

- An apparent sleep-like state.
- Highly selective attention.
- Increased suggestibility during the hypnotic state.

- Potential for post-hypnotic suggestibility.
- Increased passivity.

There is some debate as to the extent to which this state is distinct from normal suggestibility as defined above, as opposed to simply representing one extreme of a continuum of suggestibility. There is substantial anecdotal evidence of hypnotised subjects coming out of the hypnotic state when required to do something too far out of character (e.g. the anecdotal account of an assistant of Freud being slapped by a hypnotised woman he asked to pretend she was getting into bed).

Meditation and trances

A state of greatly reduced awareness of the external world, with an attendant reduction in consciousness is a *trance* state, where behaviour is reduced to the extent that the individual may appear to be asleep. This state may be self-induced, the result of religious activity, of a consequence of hypnotic induction.

Meditation may be regarded as a special case of the trance state where intense introspection is the goal. Physical and physiological correlates of such a state include:

- EEG alpha wave activity (8–12 Hz, usually found in awake, relaxed subjects).
- Lowered blood pressure and pulse.
- Lowered oxygen consumption.

Meditation is becoming increasingly popular as evidence for its therapeutic value grows (although a great many excessive claims remain unsubstantiated). Sports psychologists in particular use meditation (among other relaxation techniques) in the preparation of athletes for competition.

Summary

- *Consciousness* cannot be characterised as being simply 'on' or 'off': there are levels of consciousness, varying continuously, with some distinguishable categories (e.g. asleep versus awake). Nevertheless, while awake the level of alertness is highly variable, indicating the continuous nature of the concept. A great deal of information processing (possibly the majority) takes place without the conscious awareness of the subject, so that unconscious learning, for example, is common.
- While asleep the level of consciousness is variable also: four stages of sleep exist, distinguished primarily by the wavelength of EEG activity. A

distinct category of sleep is REM sleep, which has been closely associated with dreaming. While Freud suggested a central role for dreaming in the expression of unconscious desires, current theories suggest a cognitive restructuring function. The incidence of parasomnias is associated with specific stages of sleep.

- The existence of *periodicity* in biological functions is particularly apparent in the case of sleep, with the natural period of sleep and wakefulness being 25 hours, presumably being recalibrated daily. Sleep deprivation results in severe disruption of cognitive and motor performance after relatively little deprivation (c.12 hours).
- Altered states of consciousness, such as that achieved by *hypnosis* and *meditation* are controversial areas of research. There are certain physiological correlates of the relaxed state found in hypnotised or meditating subjects (EEG activity, blood pressure, etc.).

BASIC PSYCHOLOGY INDIVIDUAL STATEMENT QUESTIONS

The following statements are either true or false:

1. Cognitive dissonance was first described by Beck.
2. Cognitive dissonance is associated with dysphoria.
3. Cognitive dissonance predicts choices in ambiguous situations.
4. Cognitive dissonance increases with personal responsibility for action.
5. Cognitive dissonance is thought to underlie attitude formation.

6. Personal Construct Theory forms a psychodynamic understanding of personality.
7. Personal Construct Theory proposes that core constructs underlie self-identity.
8. Personal Construct Theory emphasises cognitive influences on behaviour.
9. Personal Construct Theory uses the repertory grid as a measurement tool.
10. Personal Construct Theory has been used in work on thought disorder.

11. Cognitive dissonance is specifically associated with the name of Festinger.
12. Cognitive dissonance can arise for logical reasons.
13. Cognitive dissonance results in chosen items appearing more attractive than they were before being chosen.
14. Cognitive dissonance is affectively neutral.
15. Cognitive dissonance can be reduced by dismissing or denying information.

16. Modelling can result in skilled behaviour.
17. Modelling can lower the anxiety threshold.
18. Modelling can lower the pain threshold.
19. Modelling can lead to aggression.
20. Modelling can lead to social facilitation.

21. In personality theories, Eysenck's theory is an instance of trait theory.
22. In personality theories, cognitive appraisal by the individual of their situation is excluded from consideration.
23. In personality theories, apparent stability of personality traits can be a reflection of the stability of measured intelligence.
24. In personality theories, situationism is indistinguishable from radical (traditional) behaviourism.
25. In personality theories, the causation of behaviour is of little interest to investigators compared with its description.

26. Observational learning requires vicarious satisfaction to be effective.
27. Observational learning can result in the acquisition of skills.
28. Observational learning is more likely to occur if the model has some characteristics in common with the observer.
29. Observational learning has been shown to be a mechanism whereby institutional norms of behaviour are established.
30. Observational learning is a known way of producing social inhibition.

31. In classical conditioning, an unconditioned stimulus is one that has not yet been paired with a response.
32. In classical conditioning, conditioned responses are likely to be of greater magnitude than unconditioned responses.
33. In classical conditioning, the conditioned response can recover spontaneously following extinction.
34. In classical conditioning, higher-order conditioning uses a conditioned stimulus as an unconditioned stimulus.
35. In classical conditioning, stimulus generalisation is only acquired after more than a dozen trials.

36. Perceptual constancy can be demonstrated for shape.
37. Perceptual constancy can be demonstrated for distance.
38. Perceptual constancy can be demonstrated for colour.
39. Perceptual constancy can be demonstrated for size.
40. Perceptual constancy can be demonstrated for touch.

41. According to learning theory, intermittent reinforcement schedules result in acquired behaviour that is more resistant to extinction than behaviour induced by continuous reinforcement.
42. According to learning theory, avoidance conditioning can result from a single learning trial.
43. According to learning theory, negative reinforcement means that an aversive stimulus is removed contingently on the behaviour being exhibited.
44. According to learning theory, habit strength can be estimated by the number of non-reinforced trials required to extinguish acquired behaviour.
45. According to learning theory, vicarious learning can occur even if the subject's behaviour is not reinforced.

46. Learning theory holds that avoidance conditioning is involved in the aetiology of enuresis.

47. Learning theory holds that avoidance conditioning is involved in the aetiology of exhibitionism.
48. Learning theory holds that avoidance conditioning is involved in the aetiology of agoraphobia.
49. Learning theory holds that avoidance conditioning is involved in the aetiology of obsessional rituals.
50. Learning theory holds that avoidance conditioning is involved in the aetiology of premature ejaculation.

51. A patient has gastric discomfort after eating fried food. In learning theory terms, his subsequent avoidance of fried food involves negative reinforcement.
52. A patient has gastric discomfort after eating fried food. In learning theory terms, his subsequent avoidance of fried food involves aversive training.
53. A patient has gastric discomfort after eating fried food. In learning theory terms, his subsequent avoidance of fried food involves covert sensitisation.
54. A patient has gastric discomfort after eating fried food. In learning theory terms, his subsequent avoidance of fried food involves variables reinforcement schedule.
55. A patient has gastric discomfort after eating fried food. In learning theory terms, his subsequent avoidance of fried food involves interval reinforcement schedule.

56. Free association is a concept associated with classical conditioning.
57. Chaining is a concept associated with classical conditioning.
58. Spontaneous recovery is a concept associated with classical conditioning.
59. Generalisation is a concept associated with classical conditioning stimulus.
60. Shaping is a concept associated with classical conditioning.

61. Shaping is also known as cognitive dissonance.
62. Forward chaining can be used to teach toilet training.
63. Modelling is a type of observational learning.
64. Observational learning is a form of operant conditioning.
65. A programme beginning with reinforcement of the last act in a sequence is forward chaining.

66. Operant conditioning may be understood in terms of perceptual expectancies.
67. Punishment is not synonymous with negative reinforcement.
68. Punishment results in a reduction in the probability of occurrence of a response.
69. Extinction is the process of gradual disappearance of a conditioned response on discontinuation of an unconditioned stimulus.
70. Intermittent reinforcement leads to reduced resistance to extinction than continuous reinforcement.

71. Classical conditioning takes place irrespective of the reinforcement schedule.
72. Classical conditioning takes place irrespective of the nature of the unconditioned stimulus.
73. Classical conditioning takes place irrespective of the time interval between the conditioned stimulus and the unconditioned stimulus.

74. Classical conditioning takes place irrespective of the organism's voluntary behaviour.

75. Classical conditioning takes place irrespective of the genetic potential of the organism.

76. Classical conditioning occurs most efficiently when the unconditioned stimulus precedes the conditioned stimulus.

77. Classical conditioning occurs most efficiently when the time intervals between the conditioned stimulus and the unconditioned stimulus are fixed.

78. Classical conditioning occurs most efficiently when alternative responses are available to the organism.

79. Classical conditioning occurs most efficiently when the conditioned response is strengthened by shaping.

80. Classical conditioning occurs most efficiently when the time interval between the conditioned stimulus and the unconditioned stimulus is fixed at 0.5 seconds.

81. Fixed ratio reinforcement involves reinforcing after a fixed number of correct responses.

82. Variable ratio reinforcement is at play in gambling.

83. Intermittent reinforcement takes the longest to establish.

84. Negative reinforcement can mean reinforcement via the withdrawal of unpleasant conditions.

85. Variable ratio reinforcement is the hardest to extinguish.

86. In operant conditioning, the reinforcer must affect the rate of behaviour.

87. Negative reinforcement is the removal of the aversive event.

88. In operant conditioning, the reinforcer can precede the behaviour.

89. Praise is not an effective reinforcer.

90. Negative reinforcement reduces the likelihood of a behaviour occurring.

91. Personal Construct Theory emphasises man as a historian.

92. Personal Construct Theory suggests that personality is the sum of a cluster of neurotic complexes.

93. Personal Construct Theory incorporates theories on creativity.

94. Personal Construct Theory led to the development of the repertory grid.

95. Personal Construct Theory suggests that people may sacrifice themselves to preserve core constructs.

96. Sleep during the night is mainly composed of REM sleep.

97. Sleep that includes mostly dreams is called orthodox sleep.

98. Sleep deprivation may lead to hallucinosis.

99. Sleep disorders may be associated with HLA DR2.

100. Sleep is associated with a reduction in serum growth hormone levels.

101. With regard to perception and attention, the absolute threshold is the highest intensity of a stimulus that can be tolerated.

102. With regard to perception and attention, dichotic listening can investigate selective attention.

103. With regard to perception and attention, the Stroop effect concerns rapid eye movement.
104. With regard to perception and attention, image processing beyond the primary visual cortex is usually serial processing.
105. With regard to perception and attention, top-down processing involves reading down the page.

ANSWERS

1.	F	36.	T	71.	T
2.	T	37.	F	72.	F
3.	T	38.	T	73.	F
4.	T	39.	T	74.	T
5.	F	40.	F	75.	T
6.	F	41.	T	76.	F
7.	T	42.	T	77.	F
8.	T	43.	T	78.	F
9.	T	44.	T	79.	F
10.	T	45.	T	80.	F
11.	T	46.	F	81.	T
12.	T	47.	F	82.	T
13.	T	48.	T	83.	T
14.	F	49.	T	84.	T
15.	T	50.	F	85.	T
16.	T	51.	T	86.	T
17.	T	52.	T	87.	T
18.	T	53.	F	88.	F
19.	T	54.	F	89.	F
20.	T	55.	F	90.	F
21.	T	56.	F	91.	F
22.	T	57.	F	92.	F
23.	F	58.	T	93.	T
24.	F	59.	T	94.	T
25.	T	60.	F	95.	T
26.	F	61.	F	96.	F
27.	T	62.	T	97.	F
28.	T	63.	T	98.	T
29.	T	64.	F	99.	T
30.	F	65.	F	100.	F
31.	F	66.	T	101.	F
32.	F	67.	T	102.	T
33.	T	68.	T	103.	F
34.	T	69.	T	104.	F
35.	F	70.	F	105.	F

2

Social psychology

Attitudes	63	Aggression		83
Self-psychology	68	Altruism and prosocial behaviour		86
Interpersonal psychology	69	Social psychology individual		89
Leadership	75	statement questions		
Intergroup behaviour	80			

ATTITUDES

Components

As in many cases, it is misleading to regard attitudes as a homogeneous concept. Any attitude (which may be defined in several ways but, in the field of social psychology, assumes explanatory significance rather than merely descriptive) consists of the following components:

- Cognitive — intellectual, beliefs about objects, their attributes, etc.
- Affective — most resistant to change; consists of feelings, moods, etc.
- Behavioural — pattern of behaviour related to a specific attitude.
- Conative — disposition for action related to an attitude.

In theory, these components should be highly consistent and closely related to one another, so that change in one component is correlated with change in another. In practice, however, certain components are more vulnerable to modification by situational variables (e.g. the desire to appear socially acceptable), so that behaviour may not reflect the 'true' attitude. The final, conative component is somewhat distinct.

Measurement techniques

There are three main methods by which attitudes may be assessed:

- *Thurstone scales* present items that have been rated and allocated different values. This is done by taking all items and asking a panel of appropriately selected judges to rank these according to the degree with which each item agrees with the attitude being measured (e.g. capital punishment). The subject reads the list and marks items that he or she agrees with, generating a score which reflects his/her attitude on the issue. The process of constructing such a scale is time-consuming and requires several judges in order to counter potential biases of individual judges. The overall score may mask very different responses by different subjects, measuring quantity more than quality of attitude.
- *Likert scales* differ primarily from Thurstone scales by offering subjects a range of responses on each item, usually a 5-point scale ranging from complete agreement to complete disagreement, with uncertain being the central point on the scale. Favourable and unfavourable statements are balanced to prevent response biases, for example in favour of positive responses, while the poles of the scales are alternated (i.e. complete agreement will appear first on one side and then on another) to avoid biases in the position of responses. Scoring is simply from 1 to 5 on each item and summed to achieve a total attitude score. Construction of the scale is achieved by presenting a large number of subjects with several items and then using the statistical technique of principal components analysis to select those items that appear to reflect the same dimension (i.e. attitude). This is more rapid than the construction of Thurstone scales and allows more flexibility of response, although there remains the problem of different responses resulting in the same final score and thereby masking underlying individual differences in the quality of responses.
- *Semantic differentials* give subjects the greatest freedom in response of the three methods by presenting a single line with only the poles defined by evaluative words (e.g. very dangerous to very safe). The subject places a mark at the point along the line that corresponds to the attitude held by them. Each item is scored by simply measuring the distance from one pole to the mark made by the participant, and this has to be done consistently (i.e. always from the negative end). Semantic differentials were originally designed to evaluate the meanings of individual words, but have been more frequently applied in the assessment of attitudes. Scales such as these are quick and easy to complete. Given the potential freedom of response it is encouraging from a theoretical perspective that scores tend to remain consistent over time (i.e. show good test–retest

reliability and, therefore, minimal measurement error). Unfortunately, the interpretation of moderate responses (i.e. towards the central point on the line) is problematic.

All measurement techniques are vulnerable to distortion by the desire to appear socially acceptable (political correctness, etc.), although it is possible to assess the impact of this by including some questions designed to be answered in a particular way by those attempting to present a socially acceptable image (e.g., 'Have you ever taken anything, even a paper clip, that does not belong to you?'). There is some evidence that the physiological assessment of attitudes is possible (related to polygraph/lie detector research).

Attitude change and persuasion

A great deal of research in this area has been motivated by problems of racial conflict, in particular in the USA in the 1960s. The most consistent finding, unfortunately, is that attitudes are notoriously difficult to change, to the extent that, occasionally, change in the opposite direction to that intended may occur. There are two broad methods of attitude change:

- *Incentive-based persuasion* concerns the use of reward and punishment as consequences of behaviour in order to modify this behaviour. To this extent, they focus on the behavioural components of attitudes, with the supposition that change in the other components will follow due to the underlying homogeneity of the different components of attitudes. For example, the pairing of an object with a negative stimulus may result in a negative attitude towards that object (classical conditioning) even if the pairing is not consciously noticed by the subject. Behaviour may also be modified by reinforcing the required behavioural responses (operant conditioning) to a given object.
- *Argument-based persuasion* concerns the use of information, presented in a variety of media, as a means of modifying, primarily, the cognitive and behavioural components of attitudes. The individual presenting the information, the means by which the information is passed on and the characteristics of the recipient all modify the quality and quantity of attitude change achieved. For example, certain individuals carry status that renders their advice far more powerful as a means of attitude change. This extends beyond the specific knowledge of the individuals; that is, doctors' opinions are highly regarded, with this being a general effect and not restricted to medical knowledge alone.

Several factors may modify the effectiveness of argument-based persuasion:

- The individual presenting the information:
  - Status/expertise
  - Personality/attractiveness
  - Enthusiasm
  - Non-verbal cues (eye contact, proximity)
- The means of information transmission:
  - Didactic style less effective than interactional
  - Use of fear frequently ineffective
  - Implicit message effective (requires intelligent audience)
  - Target social acceptability of attitude, not consequences

Unfortunately, while it may be possible to change an individual's overt attitude (i.e. that which is reported), behaviour and affect are far more difficult components to modify. Self-presentation and self-report biases are a consistent problem, since there is a necessary dissociation between individuals' overt attitudes (i.e. what they say) and actual attitudes (i.e. reflected in what they *do*).

Cognitive consistency and dissonance   *Festinger*

Cognitive dissonance results when two attitudes are held which are apparently inconsistent in one or more respects. A basic assumption of this concept is that this cognitive situation is untenable and individuals will spontaneously seek cognitive consistency. As such, attitudes will have to be modified or reappraised, or behaviour modified, in order for this dissonance to be reduced. An individual who does not enjoy his or her job will justify his work in other ways to reduce the dissonance created by disliking their job and yet continuing in this employment, for example by focusing on the financial rewards gained.

Consistency may be achieved intellectually, by reappraising the inconsistent attitudes in a consistent way, or behaviourally, by changing behaviour so that it becomes consistent with the attitude held. Reappraisal may include ignoring specific information or focusing on other information, or may involve seeking support for a specific pattern of beliefs.

Attitudes and behaviour

As implied above, the relationship between an attitude and subsequent behaviour is not a simple one. To a great extent, this is the result of self-presentation biases in reports of attitudes held. For example, racial prejudice is socially unacceptable, and unlikely to be admitted to by the majority, even though the actual incidence of prejudiced *behaviour* is relatively high.

In health education this divergence of apparently held beliefs and corresponding behaviour is particularly salient. An anti-smoking campaign, for example, may be effective in modifying explicit attitudes towards smoking while at the same time having little influence on smoking behaviour. To an extent, this problem may be overcome by aggregating several behavioural indicators into an overall behavioural index. Equally, a single measure of attitude is unlikely to predict a global behaviour; for example, the belief that smoking leads to lung cancer is unlikely to result in behaviour change if lung cancer is not regarded as a serious disease.

Summary

- The measurement of attitudes is notoriously difficult, being particularly vulnerable to self-presentation biases. This is further exacerbated if the attitudes being assessed are socially unacceptable (e.g. racist beliefs) or highly personal (e.g. sexual attitudes). There are three main methods of assessing attitudes: *Thurstone scales* (a list of items, which the subject may agree or disagree with, each being allocated a score); *Likert scales* (which offer a range of responses on each item); and *semantic differentials* (offering two polarised responses with a line between for the respondent to mark his/her position). Other methods have been attempted to assess attitudes (e.g. physiological apparatus similar to 'lie-detectors'), but these do not have the advantages of simplicity and cost-effectiveness of questionnaire methods.
- While it is relatively simple to change expressed attitudes (i.e. what people will admit to), it is far more difficult to change 'real' attitudes, i.e. those reflected in their behaviour towards the object of the attitude. Persuasion may be *incentive-based* (offering rewards for change) or *argument-based* (being, presumably, cheaper but more difficult). Characteristics of the individual attempting to change the subject's attitude and the means of information transmission will influence the effectiveness of such strategies. In most cases, attitudes remain particularly resistant to change, with the most consistent findings of studies in this area being negative. The attempt to frighten subjects into changing their attitudes (e.g. AIDS and condom use) is usually ineffective, while attempts to redefine social norms by making certain behaviours acceptable tend to be more successful.
- Note the four components of any attitude (cognitive, affective, behavioural and conative), again being distinct but related. It is also important to understand the role of *cognitive dissonance* as a factor influencing the justification offered by an individual for certain apparently inconsistent attitudes or related behaviours.

SELF-PSYCHOLOGY

Self-concept

In self-psychology, self-concept refers to the most complete description of an individual, and is therefore difficult to define efficiently and parsimoniously. Almost any aspect of an individual may be included in self-concept, including attitudes held about the self and others, perceived relationship with others and the environment, etc.

Broadly, self-concept may be regarded as the set of attitudes, values and beliefs that characterise the individual, or 'I'. The self-concept moderates any perception of the world and others, and consequent behaviour towards these. This may be deconstructed into related sub-concepts (see below).

Self-esteem

This refers to the degree to which one holds oneself in high regard or values oneself. It should be noted that the concept is a dimensional one, encompassing both high and low self-esteem (also known as positive and negative self-esteem, given the affective connotations of the dimension). Consequently, this is a highly evaluative concept which should be distinguished from more objective self-assessment, and low self-esteem has been associated with a wide variety of psychiatric disorders, in particular those with a strong affective component (e.g. depression, anorexia nervosa, etc.).

In contrast to the problems associated with low self-esteem, high self-esteem has been associated with a range of positive consequences and may be a protective factor, for example in the development of depression and other affective disorders. A high degree of social support and social contact is associated with high self-esteem, so that benefits become compounded, since social support and social contact are themselves protective factors.

Self-image

Related closely to self-concept, but less broad, this is a description of the self as it is imagined to be. Some have suggested that a great discrepancy between the actual self and self-image may be related to certain affective disorders. Self-image is derived from personal experiences and, importantly, the behaviour of others towards oneself. This becomes self-reinforcing, given that if one sees oneself in a certain way, one is likely to behave accordingly.

Self-recognition and personal identity

Self-recognition is understood to develop over the first 24 months of life, and is essentially the understanding of oneself as a distinct individual. For example, before the third and fourth month of life, an infant will be uninterested in his/her own reflection, or at least regard it no differently from any other reflection.

- <3rd/4th month   – little interest in own image in mirror.
- 3rd to 6th month   – reaches out to own image, but also does this for interesting toy.
- 1st year   – uses reflection to determine location of object in 'real world'.
- 18th to 24th month   – child responds to own, unusual features seen in mirror (e.g. paint).

Subsequently, the child will be able to point at his own image in the mirror and identify it: 'Me!'. The interaction of the child with a mirror, therefore, is highly revealing about the development of self-recognition. Note that a few other animals (e.g. primates) do develop a sense of self/personal identity, although the vast majority of research has concerned human subjects.

Clearly the development of a sense of the self as an individual is a fundamental requirement for the subsequent development of self-identity.

Summary

- Self-psychology, generally, refers to the conception of oneself held by an individual, in particular the *relationship* that is perceived to exist between the individual and others. The social context of self-psychology is important, as is the fact that it is the perception of the individual that is important rather than the veracity of given beliefs.
- There are two important concepts in self-psychology: the *self-concept* is the complete description of oneself held by an individual, being necessarily diffuse, difficult to define and, to an extent, fluid; a related concept is *self-esteem*, which represents the individual's sense of self-worth or value.

INTERPERSONAL PSYCHOLOGY

Person perception

The perception of ourselves and others is a central theme in social psychology, being substantially different from the perception of inanimate objects, and showing distinct and consistent biases, so that social information is processed to a great degree even before entering consciousness. The behaviour of others (and ourselves) has to be interpreted and understood, in turn leading to further inferences made from observed behaviour and other information. This information and knowledge set has to be assimilated and structured, which in turn guides subsequent inferences made from observations of behaviour.

Traditional models of person perception focus on the relationship between thoughts and cognitions regarding others and subsequent behaviour. In particular, there is substantial research focusing on the accuracy of perceptions of others, and biases which may exist in the formation of these perceptions. More recently, the influence of cognitive psychology has extended to studies of person perception in the broader context of social cognition, which is more concerned with information processing features of individual's perception of social objects (i.e. situations, others, etc.).

Affiliation

Affiliation is a broad term describing positive relationships that may vary greatly in closeness, ranging from mere co-operation to romantic love. It is not clear whether this degree of closeness represents a single continuum along which different social relationships may be characterised, or whether these social relationships vary along a range of dimensions to the extent that each should be regarded as qualitatively distinct.

Friendship

Friendship represents an important qualitative as well as quantitative difference in degree of affiliation, being a far more complex relationship than that between colleagues, for example. A number of factors influence the formation of friendships, and many of these generalise to the formation of romantic relationships also. These include:

- Physical attractiveness, which is a surprisingly important factor in the formation of friendships, and the effect is apparent even in young children. Beliefs about others are also dependent to some degree on physical attractiveness, so that, for example, attractive individuals (especially men) are regarded as more intelligent.
- Similarity, in particular of race and religion, which also improves the likelihood of friendships being formed. The importance of similarity extends beyond demographic factors such as age and social class to psychological characteristics, with personality being of particular importance. Even physical characteristics such as height have an effect.
- Mere exposure, which also appears to increase positive attitudes to others (unless a negative attitude already exists, in which case this

increases, as a result of biases in the interpretation of subsequent information to be congruent with the existing stereotype). Any object with which one is familiar is likely to elicit a positive response – this extends to works of art, music, etc.

- Proximity, which is perhaps not surprising given the importance of familiarity (above) in influencing the development of friendships. This, of course, will also be in part due to convenience and the relative proportion of acquaintances that are in close proximity.

Two theories of friendship formation have been proposed:

- The *exchange theory* argues that individuals are concerned with maximising personal gains from relationships while minimising costs; this is essentially an economic model of friendship.
- The *equity theory* argues that the primary concern is equality of costs and rewards in both partners, with evidence including the poor quality of marriages where an exchange relationship exists.

Attribution theory

An *attribution* is an explanation for behaviour (either of another or of one-self), ascribing personality characteristics, motives, beliefs, etc. on the basis of observed behaviour. This allows such behaviour to be explained and understood, and for subsequent behaviour by that individual to be predicted.

Heider proposed that the individual was a 'naïve scientist', making observations and deriving explanations and predictions on the basis of these. Heider's model, however, was not particularly scientific itself in that it did not directly generate testable hypotheses. Kelley (1967) extended Heider's original concept and suggested three types of information used to make attributions:

- Consensus   – the extent to which *others* behave in the same way.
- Consistency   – the extent to which the individual *always* behaves as such.
- Distinctiveness – the extent to which this behaviour occurs in *other* situations.

Eight possible permutations of this information are possible if each can be assigned a high or low value, and Kelley's model proposed that the permutation of information will determine the attribution made when observing a particular behaviour. For example, low consensus and distinctiveness along with high consistency should result in internal attributions. That is, if a person is the only one to behave in a specific way, does not isolate the behaviour to specific situations, and always behaves in this way, then the behaviour will be regarded as the result of an internal disposition rather than a situational factor.

Criticisms of this model concentrate on the high degree of prescriptiveness inherent in it: rather than creating a model based on observation of how individuals *do* behave, a model of how individuals *should* behave is created and observations sought to confirm this. Moreover, in most ecological (i.e. realistic) situations individuals do not choose actively to seek out such information, but instead appear to make attributions on a quite different basis (e.g. sex or age). Nevertheless, when presented with the above three types of information, a large majority of subjects make the 'correct' or predicted attributions.

Fundamental attribution error

This refers to a general tendency to overestimate the extent to which internal and stable characteristics (such as personality characteristics) motivate and cause behaviour in others, while simultaneously underestimating external and unstable (i.e. situational) factors. This tendency in the attribution of the behaviour of others has been argued to be the result of a desire to predict behaviour in others, which requires that behaviour to be the result of stable personality characteristics rather than transient situational factors. Conversely, the attribution of one's own behaviour tends to be primarily situational as opposed to dispositional, possibly because of an unwillingness to regard one's own behaviour as driven by unchanging dispositional characteristics but, instead, as a response to the contingencies present in a given situation.

Social behaviour

Attempts to understand and predict behaviour, both in others and ourselves (i.e. attributions), are central to the organisation of social interactions. Pervasive attributional biases, such as the fundamental attribution error, suggest that initial interactions will have a significant impact on subsequent interactions, the interpretation of novel information, and so on. That is, the behaviour of an individual when first met will be attributed to some internal and stable disposition, so that subsequently the same individual will be evaluated in the light of this attribution, and potentially ambiguous behaviour understood accordingly. First impressions do indeed seem to count, not least because social perceptions are modified in this way by expectations.

Stereotypes appear to be central to the process of attribution, whereby cognitive schemas suggest further attributes if one particularly salient attribute exists (e.g. the association between cultural or ethnic group and specific behavioural traits – Italians are commonly regarded as demonstrative, for example). This applies to individuals and groups and becomes self-reinforcing as congruent information is actively sought to confirm stereotypes.

'Theory of mind' in developmental disorders

A 'theory of mind' is, roughly speaking, the ability to attribute mental and intentional states to oneself and others (see Attribution theory). This allows the explanation and prediction of behaviour. In developmental psychology this is of importance in the development of imaginary play, with both inanimate objects and other peers. It has been suggested that individuals with autism lack a 'theory of mind':

- Children with autism appear to show impaired imagination.
- The impairment may be discrete, affecting only the ability to represent mental states.
- The impairment may, therefore, not affect other intellectual function.
- Functions impaired will be those that rely on mental representation (e.g. inferring behaviour).
- Social behaviour not relying on such representation will be unimpaired (e.g. greeting someone).

There is some debate as to whether the 'theory of mind' account of autism is:

- accurate, in that the results obtained which suggest a specific impairment of the ability to represent the mental states of oneself and others may be an artefact of the methodologies used; and/or
- comprehensive, in that while autistic individuals may indeed show the deficits described above this does not necessarily mean they represent the central, causal impairment.

Linguistics and interpersonal communication

An important change in the area of linguistics followed Chomsky's assertion that language is an ability that is largely genetically determined, at least in terms of its fundamental architecture, depending on the existence of specific brain structures, so that all languages share a common 'universal grammar'. That is, linguistics is not simply a description of the structure of language but tells us something about the organisation and structure of the brain and the mental processes that subserve language. A more current term is 'psycholinguistics', which emphasises the overlap between linguistics and certain elements of cognitive psychology. Main areas of interest in psycholinguistics include:

- Language acquisition.
- Second language acquisition.
- Syntax/grammar.
- Reading.
- Language and thought.
- Pragmatics (e.g. speech-act theory)

The study of *pragmatics* is of particular relevance here as this concentrates on the function of language structures in the appropriate social context, rather than on the language structure in isolation. The best example of this is the phrase 'Do you have the time?', which is clearly *not* a simple question of possession but a request. Speech-act theory is a special case of pragmatics (i.e. one particular theory) and suggests that any utterance may be construed in the context of communicating, generating behaviour in others, initiating an event, etc. Therefore, language should be regarded as an active determinant of the behaviour of the individual and others, rather than simply a consequence of behaviour. Speech acts include:

- Commissives   – making a commitment/promise.
- Declaratives   – a specific statement or declaration is made.
- Directives   – an order or request is given.
- Expressives   – no function other than social, i.e. politeness.
- Representatives – an utterance which is substituted for an action.

The development of these linguistic skills is also of interest, and appears to be primarily social and cultural. For example, expressive speech acts appear to be learned simply by repetition in children (e.g. 'What do you say?'; 'Thank you').

Summary

- The perception of the self and others differs from simple visual perception in that there is a far more central role for *attitudes*, *beliefs* and *stereotypes* to influence perceptions. Observation of others results in certain beliefs about what other attributes a given individual possesses, while existing attitudes about an individual will result in an unconscious attempt to interpret observed behaviour in a way congruent with these beliefs. Broadly similar effects exist in self-perception (cf. cognitive dissonance). The development of personal recognition and a sense of personal identity begins in the second year of life.

- *Attribution theory* relates to the explanations offered by individuals for the behaviour of themselves and others. While efforts have been made to determine what information individuals seek when attempting to make such attributions, these models tend to be prescriptive rather than descriptive. More reliably demonstrated have been the existence of *specific biases* in attributions made, with a tendency to ascribe behaviour to internal, stable characteristics in others while ascribing one's own behaviour to *environmental factors*.

- The implications of attribution include the importance of initial impressions on the subsequent behaviour of two new acquaintances, in particular since subsequent impressions will be governed by existing expectations. Several factors influence the formation of friendships, including physical attractiveness and similarity. Two theories of friendship formation and maintenance: *exchange theory* (where attempts are made to maximise personal gains while minimising costs) and *equity theory* (where a balance of costs and rewards for both individuals is sought). The extent to which these models are applicable in other relationships (e.g. family relationships, romantic affiliation, etc.) is unclear.

- The distortion of social perception, in particular the ability to ascribe mental states to oneself and others, has been suggested to be central to *autism*. This is reflected in impaired imagination and is not related to other intellectual function or social function that does not rely on internal representations (e.g. formal greetings and other tightly defined social situations with little scope for expressiveness).

- In a social context the study of *linguistics* is important when considering the role of language, which is communication and eliciting behaviour in others. The study of *pragmatics* (i.e. the function of language, rather than simply its structure and grammar) is important, including different speech acts which serve specific purposes.

LEADERSHIP

The nature of leaders

Early attempts to understand the nature of leaders, authority figures and those with group influence highlighted the role of personality factors (leaders were thought to be better educated, hold higher socioeconomic status, etc.). Many of these arguments, however, are clearly circular, since finding oneself in a position of authority will inevitably result, in most cases, in commensurate financial and social rewards.

Importantly, subsequent research showed that the characteristics of good leaders depend in part on the task in hand. For example, most groups tend to have both *task-oriented* and *emotion-oriented* leaders, with the two roles rarely being filled by the same individual. The first may be regarded as maximising productivity, for example by motivating others in the group, while the latter reduces inefficiency, for example by ensuring that the group remains happy. It is clear why it is rare for both of these roles to be fulfilled by the same individual, as they are to some degree mutually exclusive. There is also some evidence that task-oriented leaders are most important when task is highly structured, while emotion-oriented leaders best facilitate the completion of relatively unstructured tasks. Other distinctions have been made between leadership styles (as opposed to leadership *roles*):

- Democratic   – acts with support of the group and takes into account other opinions.
- Authoritarian – absolute authority, with no requirement to consult others (cf. military).
- Laissez-faire – a relaxed, informal style that promotes individuality.

The notion that certain personality traits exist in 'great' leaders is intuitively appealing, and there is some evidence that charismatic leaders are distinct (especially religious and political), but in most cases the demands of situation are also important, for example the nature of the task. For example, a democratic, emotion-centred leader would be a highly inefficient military leader. Contingency theory attempts to identify the optimal leadership style for different situations.

Social influence and social power

In broad terms, this refers to the ways in which beliefs, attitudes, opinions, behaviours, etc. in one or more others may be influenced by individuals or groups. Six methods/types of social influence have been identified:

- Rewards   – ability to confer rewards, commonly part of legitimate authority.
- Coercion   – similar to rewards, often implied in legitimate leadership roles.
- Expertise   – demonstrable expertise often useful in influencing superiors.
- Legitimacy   – influence due to status and position.
- Referential – popularity, liking, primarily by the subjects being influenced.
- Information – not necessarily conferred by position, a characteristic of the individual.

Power and obedience

Leadership implies a degree of power over others, especially in situations of authoritarian leadership. The degree of power conferred by the appointment to a certain position was illustrated famously by Milgram. Subjects, believing themselves to be taking part in a memory experiment, were all willing to administer an electric shock of at least 300 V to another 'subject' (in fact a confederate of the experimenter), with many going up to the maximum 450 V. This apparent willingness to obey orders that threaten the life of others has since been demonstrated in several countries, but falls off dramatically when there is just one other dissenting voice present, further illustrating the role of situational variables. Interestingly, the apparent authority of the experimenter could be reduced dramatically with only a *slight* reduction in the corresponding obedience of participants, for example by holding the study in an apartment flat rather than a university laboratory.

Conformity

There exists a pervasive tendency for beliefs, attitudes, etc. to be influenced by the general opinion of groups. Asch demonstrated this effect in the case of perceptual judgements where subjects tended to increase the number of false judgements of line length if several other judges have given false judgements previously. Also of interest was the observation that although in many cases subjects did insist on their own (actually correct) judgement, they did so with great apparent discomfort that they were disagreeing with the majority opinion, and often sought to justify their 'aberrant' judgement. Conformity may take the form of changes in behaviour or attitudes; changes in attitude may or may not result in corresponding behavioural change, so that the two may be regarded as essentially distinct.

Intelligence, high self-efficacy beliefs, internal locus of control are some of the internal factors which reduce the effect of conformity pressures in individuals.

Polarisation

If subjects are asked to rate their opinions on a subject individually, and then grouped and asked to reach a decision on the same subject as a group, the ultimate decision reached by the group will tend to be more extreme than the aggregated opinions of the individual group members. This effect, where an extreme opinion, in one direction or another, is reached is known as 'polarisation'. This is possibly due to the increased number of arguments in favour of a certain position available in groups, or may be due to reinforcement effects of support for one's opinion by others.

Groupthink

When a group is required to make a decision, there is a tendency for individuals to strive towards consensus (e.g. the principle of Cabinet collective accountability). The effect of this may be that individuals suppress dissenting opinions (including their own), with the consequence that flawed decisions may result if no-one is willing to speak out against them. Dissenters are censored, to the extent that individuals will suppress their own dissenting opinions, so that an impression of unanimity is achieved. Groupthink is most commonly found in the following conditions:

- High pressure for results/decisions.
- Tightly defined, cohesive group.
- Clear leader with express opinion.
- Few external influences or opinions.

The consequences of groupthink behaviour include:

- alternatives being inadequately explored;
- benefits and potential risks of preferred choice of action inadequately explored; and
- alternative/secondary/contingency choices of action not developed.

It is clear from the above that the majority of government decisions are likely to be made in groupthink conditions, and groupthink has been proposed as an explanation for decisions made by governments that, in retrospect, carried an inappropriate level of risk (e.g. the Bay of Pigs).

Deindividuation

Of particular relevance in the understanding of group behaviour is the concept of deindividuation, which is the process whereby the individuality of members of the group becomes subordinate to the behaviour of the group as a whole. Consequences of this effect include increased susceptibility to the influence of others, reduced social restraint, etc., and it can be seen in the behaviour of groups and violent mobs (cf. football crowds, riots). The effect is used to powerful effect, for example, in the use of uniforms in the armed services and prisons, where individually distinguishing features are removed and overt expressions of individuality discouraged.

Communicative control in relationships

Communicative control refers to the effect that what is said, and the structure of what is said, has on the behaviour of oneself and others (i.e. the behavioural constraints which result from patterns of speech).

In optimal relationships (whether romantic, familial, etc.), opinions and beliefs are communicated easily and readily, whereas in dysfunctional relationships this communication pattern changes and becomes damaging or destructive. Specifically, disagreement or unilaterally held beliefs may result in the use of power to resolve any conflict, rather than open communication. This may be extended to the use of disagreement as an intended precursor to the use of power or control strategies.

A significant amount of research has been carried out on the effects of communicative control in doctor–patient interactions, with the unsurprising finding that the speech and behaviour patterns of the doctor can constrain the speech and behaviour of the patient significantly.

Summary

- Leadership, social influence and social power should be distinguished. Social influence implies that the influence is in some sense earned, depending to a great extent on the characteristics of the individual, while social power implies that the obedience which results derives more from situational variables (e.g. threat, social norms for obeying certain figures, etc.). Leadership may be regarded as occupying an intermediate position, with different styles of leadership depending on either the characteristics of the individual (especially *democratic leadership*) or the situation (especially *authoritarian leadership*). This analysis is a guide rather than being prescriptive, but it illustrates that attempts to define leadership solely in terms of characteristics of individuals will be of limited value. Nevertheless, there is some evidence that 'great' leaders possess specific personality characteristics.
- When acting in groups, in particular those with a leader, certain behaviours become apparent: *polarisation* (i.e. the ultimate decision of a group will be more extreme than the individual suggestions made), *conformity* (i.e. the tendency for dissenting voices to become self-silencing) and *groupthink* (i.e. the tendency to strive for consensus, often resulting in flawed decisions).
- One should understand the role of communication in mediating group behaviour, and the extent to which speech patterns can influence the behaviour of others (cf. Pragmatics). A simple example is the use of closed, rather than open, questions, restricting the range of possible answers.

INTERGROUP BEHAVIOUR

When discussing group behaviour, one must be aware of the distinction between the *ingroup* and the *outgroup*. The ingroup is the group with which an individual identifies himself (e.g. the football team that one supports), so that any individual will be a member of several ingroups, while the outgroup is one with which the individual does not identify, whilst being one that the individual comes into contact with (e.g. a rival football team).

Prejudice

Prejudice represents the adoption of an attitude on the basis of limited or insufficient information, the implication being that the attitude is in some sense unfair or unwarranted. This strict definition implies that prejudice may be either negative or positive, whereas in reality there is a strong connotation of negativity in prejudiced attitudes (e.g. racial prejudice), which has generated a great deal of research. Prejudice relies to a great extent on the adoption of group stereotypes (see below), where a set of attributes, attitudes, etc. are imagined to apply uniformly to individual members of a specific group.

Current social cognition theories suggest that prejudice stems, at least in part, from the use of stereotypes as a means of reducing cognitive workload, facilitating ready prediction of behaviour and ascription of attitudes, etc. on the basis of limited initial information. There is also some evidence that certain individuals are more likely to adopt prejudiced attitudes on the basis of a personality disposition (authoritarianism), while others have suggested that the principal motivation behind prejudice is the disparity in beliefs and attitudes between different individuals, rather than, say, race. That is, we are attracted to those with similar beliefs and attitudes to ourselves and prejudiced against those that do not. These three models are not exclusive.

Stereotypes

As with prejudice, stereotypes in a strict sense may be positive or negative, with the central feature of stereotypes being a set of crude generalisations used to characterise members of a group. These generalisations, while being generally resistant to change, nevertheless are flexible. While consisting of generalisations, it should also be realised that these stereotypes do in fact contain an element of truth, given that they are based on some degree of information, and are *simplifications* (or generalisations) of reality rather than arbitrary constructions. As such, it is possible and meaningful to refer to the degree of accuracy that a stereotype displays.

An interesting feature of stereotypes is the extent to which highly similar stereotypes are shared by entire populations about certain groups. European nationalities, for example, tend to generate quite specific and widely shared stereotypes among Britons (and vice versa).

Stereotyping is in fact a special case of *categorisation* in a social context, being applied equally to individuals and groups. It is important to realise that once a stereotype has become established or learned, it then becomes to a degree self-fulfilling, as observations will become biased so that information which reinforces the stereotype will be sought and preferentially processed. This means that well-established stereotypes are difficult to counter (cf. prejudice).

Intergroup hostility

Minimal group experiments, where subjects are randomly assigned to membership of a group on some spurious criterion, suggest that group membership in itself (even when the randomness of group allocation is explicit), rather than the common goals, etc. usually associated with membership of a group, contributes to intergroup prejudice and conflict. In such studies subjects will, for example, preferentially allocate money to those known to be members of the same (randomly created) group, even when no other information is known (the minimal group paradigm). This suggests that intergroup behaviour is a fundamental characteristic of human (and possibly primate) social behaviour, so that there exist strong instinctive tendencies to favour preferentially *whichever* group one finds oneself a member of.

While such biases appear even when there is no direct competition for resources, overt hostility is usually associated with some sort of direct competition. Several studies of group behaviour have demonstrated that as soon as competition for resources becomes a feature of intergroup transactions, some level of hostility is usual. The situation is more complex because certain intergroup transactions imply a certain level of hostility – for example, between prison warders and inmates. In this case it is problematic to speak of competition for resources. There is also evidence that the absolute level of resources attained by a group is of less importance than the relative *superiority* over a competing group in the allocation of resources. That is, groups will choose to attain less resources as long as the level attained is greater than that attained by a competing group.

Social identity and group membership

Membership of a group is associated with certain effects on social perception, with clear biases evident. For example:

- Ingroup rated as more heterogeneous (cf. fundamental attribution error).
- Outgroup rated as more homogeneous (cf. fundamental attribution error).
- This is reversed if the ingroup is the minority group (maintain group identity).
- Ingroup members rated more positively (self-esteem?).

Membership of groups is a significant factor in defining social identity, with the effect being even stronger in less individualistic (e.g. Eastern) cultures. Intergroup discrimination and prejudice is related to elevated self-esteem in the group displaying prejudice, and may be explained by the need to achieve a clear social identity, given that this confers a sense of self-esteem. Therefore, the more distinctive the ingroup becomes, the greater the self-esteem of ingroup members, and this may be achieved by group-serving biases and perceived outgroup homogeneity (stereotyping). This perceived outgroup homogeneity may be related to the attribution of behaviour to dispositional characteristics in individual judgements (and the converse attribution of ones own behaviour to situational characteristics, which may correspond to the tendency to regard the ingroup as relatively heterogeneous).

Summary

- It is important to understand the use of *ingroup* and *outgroup* to define those who do and do not belong to a specific group (being a necessarily relative term), as well as the fact that most individuals will identify with a number of groups of varying order (e.g. nationality, social class, etc.).
- The information processing biases, attributions, stereotypes and schemata found in individual social perception extend to *group behaviour*, so that the group can be roughly substituted for the individual and similar effects expected. Note that while prejudice and stereotype implies a certain degree of negativity, although in principle these may be positive or negative, with the important component of these being a degree of cognitive parsimony (i.e. basing conclusions on limited or insufficient information).
- Minimal group experiments (where subjects are assigned to a group on random criteria) suggest that membership of a group results in a degree of *hostility* towards those identified as belonging to the outgroup, even in cases where there is no direct competition for resources.
- The benefits of group membership can be seen in the role groups play in defining an individual's social identity, even in individualistic, Western cultures, being related to positive self-esteem.

AGGRESSION

Aggression is a very general term for any action or behaviour that displays a degree of hostility, and is predictably difficult to define. Comparisons across studies should, therefore, be cautious. Motivations for aggressive behaviour may include:

- Desire to gain resources (including winning an argument).
- Desire to intimidate others.
- A reaction to intimidation by others.

Given the number of possible motivating factors and definitions of aggression, there exist several theories by which it may be explained.

Social learning theory

By a process of modelling it is suggested that the majority of behaviours, including aggressive behaviours, are learned at an early age, through observation of parents initially and then other salient figures (peers, teachers, media personalities, etc.). Observation of aggressive behaviour and its consequences in others will result in such behaviour being imitated by the observer. Experimental evidence is strong: children who observe an adult striking an inflatable doll are more likely to do so themselves when the opportunity arises than children who observe an adult acting neutrally towards the doll. Importantly, this effect remains if the observation is via video, with obvious implications for the effect of television on aggressive behaviour.

Operant conditioning

Given that aggressive behaviour may be seen as a means of achieving goals, the consequences of aggressive behaviour will be important in determining whether such behaviour is likely to occur again. That is, in an operant conditioning model, the consequences of aggressive behaviour may be reinforcing, and may include gaining resources and objects (physical reinforcement) or gaining social approval (social reinforcement). Social learning theories of aggressive behaviour may be regarded as vicarious (i.e. observational) operant conditioning models.

Ethology

Ethological theories suggest that aggression is an instinctive behaviour, serving an adaptive function promoting the survival of genes that confer aggressive behaviour (i.e. natural selection). Aggression between species serves to ensure the survival of the more aggressive group, since this group will achieve more resources at the expense of other species (groups). Within-species aggression allows hierarchies to be established and ensures that within-species groups remain at optimal size and do not come into competition for resources.

Therefore, aggression is an instinctive behaviour that, while being dependent to a degree on situational factors, is nevertheless ultimately inevitable. After an aggressive act the 'potential' for further aggression decreases, gradually increasing again until the next aggressive act.

Frustration

The frustration–aggression hypothesis suggests that frustration and aggression are intimately linked, so that frustration (i.e. the inability to attain a desired goal) always leads to some form of aggression (although not necessarily overt), while aggression is always the result of some prior frustration.

Frustration is suggested to arise primarily from failure to achieve goals, which induces a drive towards frustration. The aggressive behaviour need not be directed towards the cause of the frustration, and indeed need not even be overt (displacement). While intuitively appealing, this hypothesis suffers from problems of circularity. Furthermore, frustration may also lead to behaviours such as apathy (depression?) or emotional distress, rather than aggression. These last objections have led to a minor reformulation of the theory, weakening the causal link between frustration and aggression so that aggression is regarded as the most likely response, rather than the only possible response.

Arousal

If the frustration–aggression hypothesis (see above) is modified to weaken the causal link between frustration and aggression it becomes somewhat impoverished, and the question of what causes aggression remains. This may be accounted for by suggesting that specific environmental cues result in existing frustration being translated into aggressive behaviour. By a process of classical conditioning these environmental cues will have become associated with aggressive behaviour, anger, and so on. This allows for situational variables to be accounted for, whereas the frustration–aggression hypothesis relies almost entirely on internal factors. There is some experimental evidence that the presence of aggression-congruent cues results in increased aggressive behaviour in angry (i.e. frustrated) subjects.

Media influences

There is substantial current interest in the question of whether violence and aggressive behaviour generally, as seen in the media (especially on television and in films), has an influence on the behaviour of observers, particularly in children. Certainly, social learning models of aggression would suggest a very strong link between the portrayal of violence and the performance of violence by observers. Several longitudinal studies confirm this, suggesting a significant correlation between violent material watched on television, for example, and incidence of aggressive behaviour. The effect extends beyond aggressive behaviour and appears to influence attitudes towards aggression and violence (cognitive dissonance?).

The effect is not as simple as it may first appear, however: there is some evidence that the effect exists, or at least is strongest, in those with a predisposition to aggressive behaviour initially. This suggests that there are also individual differences in aggression that interact with situational variables.

Aggressive individuals

The development of aggressive behaviour is highly complex, but there are certain correlates, such that the following factors have been shown, with varying degrees of support, to be related to aggressive behaviour in individuals:

- Aggressive parents.
- The use of physical punishment by parents.
- Young parents.
- Lower socioeconomic status.
- Large family size.
- Lack of positive emotional expression in the family.
- Highly permissive or inconsistent parenting styles.

Clearly more factors could be added to this list, and those on it are subject to some debate. It is also very important to distinguish between correlation (as in these cases), and causation (which is *not* necessarily implied). Nevertheless, the parenting style adopted by parents will have a strong influence on the subsequent behaviour of the child, and the behaviour of parents will in part be determined by situational and environmental constraints (e.g. large family size results in less time with each child).

Summary

- Several theories of *aggression* exist: social learning theory (i.e. behaviours are observed in significant others and modelled), operant conditioning (i.e. aggressive behaviour results in goals being achieved, which is positively reinforcing), ethological theory (i.e. aggression is an instinctive behaviour which serves an adaptive purpose in evolutionary terms), frustration–aggression hypothesis (i.e. failure to achieve goals results in frustration, which may be resolved by aggression), and arousal theory (i.e. certain environmental cues become associated with aggression, serving to increase the likelihood of this).
- The current debate on the role of the media in influencing *violent behaviour*, especially in children, may draw on this literature. In particular, social learning theory suggests that the observation of violent behaviour will result in this behaviour being imitated (modelled).
- It is possible (indeed likely) that several theories will be correct. For example, social learning theory has difficulty accounting for the range of individual differences in aggressive behaviour. Several factors have been shown to be related to aggressive behaviour.

ALTRUISM AND PROSOCIAL BEHAVIOUR

Altruism

Generally, this is used to describe helping behaviour where the interests of others are favoured over the interests of self. Strictly, altruistic behaviour should not include any component that may be regarded as beneficial for the individual performing the act. In this sense, there is some debate as to whether truly altruistic behaviour may be said to exist at all, given that it is always possible to ascribe some selfish (possibly unconscious) motivation behind apparently altruistic behaviour, such as a consequent elevation of self-esteem, a sense of well-being, etc. It is important, therefore, to distinguish between altruism, as defined above, and *helping behaviour*, where there is no requirement for the action to be entirely unselfish. Certainly, helping behaviour generally is far more common than apparent instances of true altruism.

In ethology and evolutionary biology, certain apparently altruistic behaviours present paradoxes, such as the alarm signal of some birds, which warns other members of the group but puts the individual at increased risk of harm. In such cases it is possible to hypothesise an evolutionary advantage conferred by such behaviour, so that natural selection will make such behaviour likely. The genetic correlates of this alarm signal behaviour, for example, will be shared by other members of the species, so that the behaviour serves to promote the survival of those genetic correlates (if not the individual bird itself).

Social exchange theory

As a general model of social behaviour, social exchange theory suggests that behaviour is motivated by the expectation that such behaviour will result in some form of reward from others. Consequently, helping behaviour is motivated by the hope that if the individual were in need of help, then others would act similarly. This model is also amenable to evolutionary explanation or interpretation. It may be regarded as an economic model, with the individual taking into account the costs and potential rewards of any given behaviour (again, not necessarily consciously).

Helping relationships

Several factors influence whether helping behaviour is likely:

- Social responsibility norms.
- Personal or individual norms.
- Reciprocity norms.
- High self-efficacy beliefs/confidence in ability to help.

Other factors reduce the likelihood of helping behaviour:

- Bystander effect/diffusion of responsibility.
- Low self-efficacy beliefs/subjective inability to help.
- Uncertainty of situation/ambiguity.

These factors explain cases of passivity or lack of helping behaviour that are at least as common as cases of heroism and helping behaviour in highly dangerous situations. The bystander effect is commonly cited (cf. the celebrated Kitty Genovese case, where almost 40 individuals observed and failed to report an attack), but poorly understood.

Interpersonal co-operation

Co-operative behaviours are apparent between individuals and between groups, and results are broadly generalisable. In the majority of cases, co-operation stems from situations where a goal is unattainable by the individual or group alone, and the assistance of another individual or group who desires the same goal is required. This necessarily requires the goal to be one that can be shared. In such cases, intergroup or interpersonal conflict, prejudice, negative attitudes, etc. may be greatly reduced, and this is perhaps the only reliable means of reducing conflict between groups.

The 'prisoner's dilemma' is an experimental device to study the pattern of co-operation between two individuals, where a choice has to be made which determines one's outcome, but which also determines the outcome for another individual (and vice versa). The two subjects are given choices for action where, if both choose the same action the reward is greatest, but the risk is also greatest if the other chooses a different action. For example, if both choose A, each wins £5; however, if subject 1 chooses A and subject 2 chooses B, the reward for subject 2 is £6 and the reward for subject 1 is £1. If both choose B, the reward is £3.

Several factors influence co-operative behaviour:

- Number of individuals (low co-operation in large groups).
- Behaviour of other individual(s).
- Potential costs and benefits of specific actions.
- Degree of communication.
- Previous knowledge of other individual(s).

Summary

- One should distinguish between *altruism* (defined as behaviour where the interests of other is elevated above the interests of oneself, so that there is no personal gain), *helping behaviour* (where helping behaviour takes place but there may also be some gain for the individual offering the help) and *prosocial behaviour* (which refers to positive social behaviour in general). Altruism is often conflated, mistakenly, with helping behaviour more generally.
- Several factors influence the likelihood of helping behaviour taking place (e.g. social norms, individual norms, expectation of reward), while others reduce this likelihood (e.g. bystander effect, low self-efficacy beliefs). It is difficult to suggest that 'true' altruism (as defined above) exists as it is always possible to infer a gain for the helping individual (e.g. elevated self-esteem). Exchange theory (see page 87) has been suggested to be useful in understanding helping behaviour, so that the likelihood of helping behaviour occurring will in part be the result of potential gains versus potential costs.
- Co-operation may be regarded as a special case of helping behaviour where a goal may only be achieved if two individuals work together. In this case there is no clear 'giver' or 'receiver' of help, except in the sense that both individuals (or groups) carry out both roles. Familiarity and good communication increases the likelihood of co-operation, while large groups tend to result in low levels of co-operation.

SOCIAL PSYCHOLOGY INDIVIDUAL STATEMENT QUESTIONS

The following statements are either true or false:

1. In expressing judgements about visual measurements, an individual will usually change their decision if the group they are in expresses a contrary opinion.
2. In expressing judgements about visual measurements, a unanimous group of 20 is much more likely than a unanimous group of three to persuade an individual to change his or her decision.
3. In expressing judgements about visual measurements, an individual is far less likely to yield to a group decision if just one other individual agrees with him or her.
4. In expressing judgements about visual measurements, the majority of individuals will stick to their own opinion in the face of group opposition.
5. In expressing judgements about visual measurements, an individual can easily persuade a group to change their group opinion.

6. Aggressive behaviour may be conceptualised in behavioural terms using reaction forming.
7. Aggressive behaviour may be conceptualised in behavioural terms using operant conditioning.
8. Aggressive behaviour may be conceptualised in behavioural terms using classical conditioning.
9. Aggressive behaviour may be conceptualised in behavioural terms using stimulus fading.
10. Aggressive behaviour may be conceptualised in behavioural terms using modelling.

11. Friendship is increased by proximity.
12. Friendship is increased by being complimentary more than by similarity.
13. Friendship is increased by reciprocal disclosure.
14. Friendship is increased by familiarity.
15. Friendship is increased by physical attractiveness.

16. In the measurement of attitudes the results obtained on a recognised test will usually be a good predictor of behaviour across social situations.
17. In the measurement of attitudes, Likert scales use a multiple choice format.
18. In the measurement of attitudes, visual analogue scales are prone to a positional response set.
19. In the measurement of attitudes, a Thurstone scale requires the subject to select one statement from a range of options.
20. In the measurement of attitudes, semantic differential scales have the advantage of immunity from social desirability.

21. Vulnerability of an individual to group pressure to change his/her mind increases with intelligence.
22. Vulnerability of an individual to group pressure to change his/her mind increases in a linear fashion with the number of opponents.
23. Vulnerability of an individual to group pressure to change his/her mind results from a mathematical sum of supporting and opposing individuals.
24. Vulnerability of an individual to group pressure to change his/her mind decreases with global social effectiveness.
25. Vulnerability of an individual to group pressure to change his/her mind was studied by Asch.

26. Concerning attitudes the belief components correlate very highly with the behavioural components.
27. Concerning attitudes changes in beliefs may be provoked by cognitive dissonance.
28. Concerning attitudes first impressions of other people are governed more by dispositional rather than situational attributions.
29. Concerning attitudes assessment by Likert scaling requires the subject to indicate responses to items on a 5-point scale of agreement.
30. Concerning attitudes the affective component is closely linked with moral approval or disapproval.

31. Studies of small groups have shown members' original individual judgements of line length to be distorted by the opinions of others in that group.
32. Studies of small groups have shown conformity to be greater in groups with high cohesiveness.
33. Studies of small groups have shown the group setting affects the risk-taking decision by individuals.
34. Studies of small groups have shown that both informational and normative social influences can lead to individual members changing their original decisions.
35. Studies of small groups have shown the group setting affects moral choices.

ANSWERS

1. T	**13.** T	**25.** T
2. F	**14.** T	**26.** F
3. T	**15.** F	**27.** T
4. F	**16.** F	**28.** T
5. F	**17.** T	**29.** T
6. F	**18.** T	**30.** T
7. T	**19.** T	**31.** T
8. F	**20.** F	**32.** T
9. F	**21.** F	**33.** T
10. T	**22.** F	**34.** T
11. T	**23.** F	**35.** T
12. F	**24.** T	

3

Neuropsychology

Brain organisation   93   Neuropsychology individual   99
                                        statement questions

BRAIN ORGANISATION

The underpinning assumption of human neuropsychology is that all behaviour is a reflection of brain function. To this end, modification of brain function (either carried out on purpose or resulting from accidental damage) should result in a change in behaviour, which in turn will suggest the localised function of the corresponding area of the brain. Several techniques are employed:

- Brain damage/surgery
- Electroencephalography (EEG)
- Event-related potential (ERP)
- Magnetoencephalography (MEG)
- Computed axial tomography (CAT/CT)
- Positron emission tomography (PET)
- Functional magnetic resonance imaging (fMRI)
- Biochemical techniques
- Brain electrical stimulation
- Lateralisation techniques

These techniques all share the common feature that they in some way modify (through inhibition or stimulation) the function of a localised area of the brain (e.g. brain damage, brain electrical stimulation), or provide information as to the differential degree of activity in brain regions during a period of specified behaviour (e.g. PET, fMRI).

Memory

Much of the evidence implicating particular regions of the brain in the function of memory comes from pathological memory, usually resulting from brain damage:

- Amnesia   –   a partial or total loss of memory
- Retrograde amnesia   –   difficulty recalling events prior to the onset of amnesia
- Anterograde amnesia   –   difficulty recalling events subsequent to the onset of amnesia

Unlike many other abilities or functions, memory does not appear to be highly localised in the brain. For example, memory impairment in rats appears to be more closely related to the total amount of cortex removed, rather than to the specific location of the lesion. Nevertheless, stimulation of highly localised areas of the cortex in humans elicits specific memories, suggesting that specific memories are localised, while memory in general may not be. The question is very far from being adequately resolved, but there is evidence for some localisation of memory.

Some evidence suggests that encoding and retrieval functions are dissociated, as is long-term and short-term memory:

- Left hemisphere most active during encoding.
- Right hemisphere most active during retrieval.

Furthermore, these different functions may, to some degree, be localised. Lesion studies in humans have provided strong evidence for the dissociation of short-term and long-term memory, with some patients showing intact short-term and long-term memory but an inability to transfer *new* information from the former to the latter.

Damage to the temporal lobe (in particular the anterior temporal cortex, the amygdala, the hippocampus and the entorhinal cortex) is associated with various degrees of amnesia. Also, damage to either of the major structures of the diencephalons (the hypothalamus and the thalamus) causes amnesia, both of which become degenerated to some degree in chronic alcoholics who display Korsakoff's syndrome. Finally, damage to the basal forebrain (consisting of the nucleus accumbens, spetal nuclei, anterior hypothalamus, nucleus of Meynert and the prefrontal cortex) is associated with memory impairment. In particular, the prefrontal cortex appears especially important for working memory.

Language

Invasive and non-invasive studies of localisation have shown left hemisphere dominance for speech and language. Electrical stimulation studies, for example, report impaired speech following left-sided but not right-sided stimulation. Two regions of the (almost exclusively) left hemisphere appear critical for language:

- *Broca's area*: this is located in inferior frontal gyrus. Damage to this area results in loss of speech fluidity and severely deficient syntax, suggesting that the area plays a role in the production of grammatically correct sentences. These deficits (impaired speech production and syntax) generalise to written language, but comprehension of both spoken and written language may be unimpaired.
- *Wernicke's area*: this is a less well-defined area in the frontal region. In subjects with damage to this area speech production is fluid and syntactically correct. The use of specific words, however, is often impaired, so that neologisms, related words ('knife' instead of 'fork') or entirely inappropriate words may be used, as well as imprecise words ('thing').

While Broca's and Wernicke's areas have received the greatest attention, it is inappropriate to regard these as the primary language areas, as a number of other areas are related to language function. Brain-damaged patients frequently provide insights into the function which are to some degree localised or dissociated, such that only one specific function is impaired.

It should be noted that, in adults, damage to a primary language area results in permanent deficit. In children before the age of 7–8 years, with language already intact, such damage results in temporary deficit, with function returning after several months or a few years. In young, pre-linguistic children gross damage to the left hemisphere does not result in subsequent linguistic deficit, and language develops normally, suggesting that the left hemisphere is not unique in the ability to sustain linguistic ability, even if this is the normal site of development. There is also some evidence that the right hemisphere does play some part in language processing, in particular if the verbal task is automatic (such as reciting the days of the week). The right hemisphere is also active during the comprehension of metaphors (possibly due to the role of the right hemisphere in mental imagery), and in the processing of the affective tone of speech.

Three principal language disorders exist:

- *Aphasia*, which is a disturbance in the comprehension or production of speech.
- *Dysgraphia*, which is an impairment in the production of written language.
- *Dyslexia*, which is an impairment in the comprehension or reading of written language.

Characteristics and primary symptoms of these conditions are listed in Table 3.1.

Table 3.1 *Characteristics and primary symptoms of aphasia, dysgraphia and dyslexia*

Condition	Primary symptoms
Aphasias	
Sensory (Wernicke's) aphasia	General comprehension deficits, neologisms, word retrieval deficits, semantic paraphasias
Production (Broca's) aphasia	Speech production deficits, abnormal prosody, impaired syntactic comprehension
Conduction aphasia	Naming deficits and impaired ability to repeat non-meaningful single words and word strings
Deep dysphasia	Word repetition deficits, verbal (semantic) paraphasia
Transcortical sensory aphasia	Impaired comprehension, naming, reading and writing, semantic irrelevancies in speech
Transcortical motor aphasia	Transient mutism and telegrammatic, dysprosodic speech
Global aphasia	Generalised deficits in comprehension, repetition, naming and speech production
Dysgraphias	
Phonological agraphia	Deficient spelling of non-words, real words spelled 'visually'
Orthographic (surface) dysgraphia	Impaired spelling of irregular words, regular words and non-words spelled phonetically
Deep agraphia	Inability to spell phonetically, tendency to make semantic substitutions
Dyslexias	
Visual word form dyslexia	Impaired sight reading, some decoding is possible
Phonological dyslexia	Deficits in reading pseudowords and non-words
Surface dyslexia	Produce regularisation errors in reading of irregular words
Deep dyslexia	Semantic substitutions, impaired reading of abstract words, inability to read non-words
Developmental dyslexia	Impaired reading and spelling of words, non-words and pseudowords, some visuoperceptual deficits

Perception

Sensory projection areas are those regions of the cortex that receive sensory information. Electrical stimulation of specific areas results in corresponding sensations. The areas are specified by the sensory modality that is served by that area (visual, somatosensory, etc.).

- The *somatosensory area*: this is located in the parietal lobes. Stimulation of this area results in sensations of tingling, warmth, cold, etc.
- The *visual area*: this is located in the occipital lobes. Stimulation here results in visual experience, but with no form or real content (e.g. flickering lights).
- The *auditory area*: this is located in the temporal lobes. As with the visual area, stimulation results in auditory experiences that are meaningless.

Three broad categories of perceptual disorder include:

- *Agnosia*, which is the inability to recognise objects in any sensory modality despite intact sensory apparatus. Colour agnosia refers to the inability to name colours, despite being able to discriminate between them. Prosopagnosia is the inability to recognise individual faces.
- *Blindsight*, which describes the ability of patients with striatal cortex damage and who are therefore cortically blind to complete perceptual tasks successfully despite self-reports of being unaware of stimuli being presented.
- *Spatial neglect*, which describes the inability to attend to stimuli in one hemifield (usually left, where the condition is more severe), resulting from damage to the opposing (i.e. usually right) parietotemporal area.

Visuospatial ability

Visuospatial ability appears to be more reliant on the performance of the right than the left hemisphere. The visual area of the brain (located in the occipital lobes) may be further divided into that area which is responsible for the recognition of stimuli and that area which is responsible for the localisation in space of stimuli. The following fundamental perceptual abilities are located in broadly the same area of the visual cortex:

- object segregation;
- distance perception; and
- movement perception.

Again, lesion studies have provided evidence for the localisation and dissociation of these functions, with patients showing quite distinct and well-defined deficits. A division has been suggested between tests of spatial transformation (such as mental rotation ability), which do appear to elicit reliable hemispheric asymmetries, and tests involving spatial relations (such as categorising objects as 'outside of' or 'above'). Right posterior brain damage is associated with mental rotation deficit, whereas a left visual field advantage is found for mental rotation in healthy individuals. Other visuospatial, right-hemisphere functions include the perception and recognition of non-verbal visual stimuli such as faces. Spatial processing is not limited exclusively to the right hemisphere, however, and visuospatial deficits have been reported in patients with left-hemisphere lesions. Clarification of the type of visuospatial test used is crucial in determining the type of localisation.

Frontal lobe functions

The frontal lobes comprise about one-third of the human neocortex, and in evolutionary terms are the most recent part of the cerebrum. Their principal roles are associated with higher mental functions, in particular the modulation of emotional responses and emotional memories, the association of these with current behaviour, and the planning and maintenance of goals. These are called 'executive functions'. The frontal lobes are also thought to regulate social behaviour and regulate and plan voluntary movement (as they contain the premotor cortex).

The frontal lobes in general play very little part in receiving direct sensory information, and instead serve to integrate information from other, primary receptive areas of the brain via association cortices. There are also selective connections with the limbic system. The integration takes the form of both assimilating information from various sensory modalities, and of integrating this information with past experience and emotional responses. As such, the frontal lobes are said to perform a largely associative function.

Given the role of the frontal lobes in modulating (and moderating) emotional responses, surgical intervention in cases of manic-depression has been performed since the 1930s. Unfortunately, this procedure is largely unsuccessful, and any benefits that do result tend to be countered by considerable side effects (blunted affect, apathy, seizures, etc.). This psychosurgical procedure has also been used in cases of chronic pain, with a similar lack of success.

Frontal lobe damage produces motor (precentral) and cognitive (prefrontal) symptoms. Not all frontal lobe patients exhibit the same or all of these symptoms. *Motor symptoms* include an inability to make voluntary motor (limb) movements or voluntary eye movements. *Cognitive symptoms* include an inability to behave spontaneously, plan and form strategies, execute strategies effectively, shift strategies and maintain attention. Other cognitive symptoms include poor free memory recall and impaired working memory. Frontal lobe damage is also associated with changes in affect, personality and social behaviour.

Summary

- Memory appears to be diffused through the brain, rather than highly localised, although there is evidence for hemispheric specialisation in encoding and retrieval.
- Most research on language function in the brain has focused on two regions: *Broca's area* (which is responsible for grammatical accuracy and syntax) and *Wernicke's area* (which is responsible for the semantic content of sentences).
- *Perception* is further localised according to the modality of the sense, with evidence for separate somatosensory, visual and auditory areas.
- The *frontal lobes* are generally associated with higher-level mental functions, in particular the modulation of emotional responses and the co-ordination of information from other regions, in particular the various perceptual areas (above).

NEUROPSYCHOLOGY INDIVIDUAL STATEMENT QUESTIONS

The following statements are either true or false:

1. Retrograde amnesia refers to amnesia where the difficulty in recalling events becomes more severe over time.
2. Anterograde amnesia refers to difficulty or impairment in recalling events that have happened after the onset of amnesia.
3. Damage to Broca's area is associated with deficits in the production of spoken language, but not written language.
4. Damage to Broca's area may still leave the comprehension of spoken and written language intact.
5. In agnosia the sensory apparatus is intact, but the ability to recognise objects is impaired.

6. In colour agnosia the ability to discriminate between colours is impaired.
7. The frontal lobes are associated with the control of emotional responses.

ANSWERS

1. F
2. T
3. F
4. T
5. T
6. F
7. T

Psychological assessment

Principles of measurement   101   Psychological assessment   112
Intelligence   105   individual statement questions
Neuropsychological assessment   109

PRINCIPLES OF MEASUREMENT

The characteristics of a good test/assessment tool include:

- Discriminatory power
- Standardised scores
- Reliability
- Validity

The *reliability* of a test reflects the extent to which a test will produce replicable results, and is a measurement of the contribution of random error to the observed value, given that any observed value will consist of the true value plus both random and systematic error. For example, a good ruler will measure the same distance as, say, a centimetre every time. A ruler that expanded or contracted with slight changes in temperature would be highly unreliable (random error), although a ruler that included 11 millimetres in every centimetre (systematic error) would still be reliable (although it would not be a *valid* measure of centimetres). In the same way, a psychometric test that gave varying results as the situation changed would display poor reliability. Therefore, psychometric instruments must be designed to minimise the impact of random error. There are five main tests of reliability:

- Test–retest reliability   – correlation of scores at two different test times.
- Alternate form reliability – correlation of two different forms of the test.

- Split-half reliability   – correlation of first half of test score with second half.
- Cronbach's alpha   – the aggregate of all possible split-halves of a test.
- Inter-rater reliability   – correlation of scores produced by two raters.

Validity represents the degree to which a test measures something meaningful, specifically what it is intended to measure. For example, do IQ scores genuinely reflect some underlying, global intellectual capacity, or simply cultural competence? Four forms of validity are:

- Criterion validity: correlation of test score with external criterion (and may be predictive or concurrent).
- Construct validity: relationship of test to underlying construct, for example intelligence (and may be convergent or discriminant).
- Face validity: degree to which items appear salient and relevant given the overt purpose of the test.
- Content validity: degree to which test items are a broad and representative selection of the items related to the concept/construct being tested.

Scaling

A *scale* may be regarded as a tool for placing items or objects in a particular order on the basis of some criterion. For example, individuals may be ordered by height or weight, with the score on the scale reflecting some underlying property. Four main types of scale exist:

- *Nominal scales* are very simple, qualitative classificatory systems for the grouping of observations, and are not amenable to statistical analysis. An example would be the classification of psychiatric conditions.
- *Ordinal scales* are those where position on the scale represents a relative value so that, for example, a higher score represents 'more' of a certain property. Here it is relative, rather than absolute, value that is measured, An example might be happiness, scored from 1 to 7.
- *Interval scales* differ from ordinal scales in that the differences between scores are precise and equal. Temperature scales, for example, assume that the difference between 30°C and 40°C is equal to the difference between 80°C and 90°C.
- *Ratio scales* differ from interval scales in that a zero value reflects a complete lack of the given property. Weight is such a scale, as zero weight reflects a complete lack of that property. Temperature, therefore, is an interval scale unless measured in Kelvin, where an absolute zero exists.

The construction of a scale, and its use, is scaling, with the scaling of psychological (i.e. subjective) properties presenting unique problems not present in the physical sciences. Some question the validity of applying statistical methods and quantitative measurement of such properties, although it is these means that represent psychology's objective and scientific basis.

Psychological (or psychometric) assessment tools should be distinguished from psychophysical assessment tools. The latter measure some characteristic that has a direct physical correlate (e.g. perceived temperature), while the former measure constructs that do not have such direct correlates (e.g. intelligence, emotion).

Ratios

A general definition of ratio would be that it is the relative magnitude of two scores, so that intelligence quotient, for example, was originally scored as intellectual age divided by chronological age (a now redundant usage).

It should be noted that many scores are in fact misclassified as ratio or interval scores, on the assumption that the interval units are comparable and the distribution of scores normal. IQ scores are usually treated (inappropriately) in this way as it allows for more powerful statistical analysis.

Norm-referenced approaches

The primary function of psychological assessment tests and tools is to allow comparison of individuals along one or more dimensions. While it may be useful to compare subjects within a study, this approach is limited since results from such studies cannot be readily generalised. To this end, it may be necessary to make an external comparison of all subjects within a study to determine whether they differ significantly from the normal population. Consequently, the majority of well-established tests provide population norms for the dimensions measured by the test.

IQ tests, for example, are designed such that the distribution of scores within the intended population will be normal, with a mean of 100. The norms for personality scales such as the Eysenck Personality Questionnaire represent another example, in this case being divided into sub-populations (e.g. by age group or occupation). While such approaches allow for detailed comparison of scores and the application of powerful statistical methods, the process of obtaining such norms is necessarily time-consuming and expensive.

It is common, although not required, for scores which lie more than one standard deviation from the norm to be regarded as distinct if classification of subjects is required. For example, if a comparison of subjects is required on the basis of intelligence it may be simplest to compare high, low and moderate intelligence groups, so that cut-off scores are required for each category.

Criterion-referenced approaches

There are several means by which a score on a test may be compared with some criterion score. Generally, this approach allows for the comparison of individuals against a standard, from which interpretations may be drawn. This standard may be set relatively simply (in contrast to norm-referenced approaches – see above), and is particularly valuable in assessing changes in performance over time of progress. In psychophysical studies, for example, the criterion for non-detection of a stimulus may be a specific period where the probability of detection is only 0.5 (50%).

In the case of more subjective attributes the criterion may be established by means of a criterion group, where a selection of representative individuals is scored using the same means to provide a comparison score for other individuals. A test of artistic ability, for example, may be administered to a group of painters in order to provide the test with some internal (construct) validity. This may also allow for cut-off scores to be established: a test designed to assess depression in subjects may require a cut-off score above which subjects are regarded as clinical cases (e.g. Hospital Anxiety and Depression scale), and this may be established by means of a criterion group.

Summary

- The two most important features of any test are its *reliability* and *validity*. Reliability may be assessed in several ways: test–retest (where the correlation of scores over time is assessed); alternative form (where the scores of different tests of the same ability are correlated); and split-half (where the sub-score on half of the test is correlated with the score on the other half). Validity takes different forms: criterion, construct, face and concurrent are the most important.
- Different types of *scale* exist: nominal, ordinal, interval and ratio. The properties of each of these includes, most importantly, the type of statistical operations which may be carried, determined in part by the assumption on which the scale rests (e.g. a normal distribution of scores in a given population).
- Two different approaches should be understood: *norm-referenced* and *criterion-referenced*. Norm-referenced approaches either define (e.g. IQ) or assess (e.g. personality) the norm for a population, allowing individuals to be compared to this. Criterion-referenced approaches compare the score of an individual on a test with some criterion (e.g. a 50% probability of detecting a stimulus in psychophysical tasks).

INTELLIGENCE

Definitions

Definitions of intelligence are various, and no one satisfactory definition exists. Instead, it is best to define intelligence in a specific way, outlining what is being sought and how this will be done. There are several potential approaches:

- Psychometric   – the delineation of specific and general abilities.
- Computational – the information-processing correlated with psychometric abilities.
- Biological   – the neural and physiological correlates of above two approaches.
- Developmental – interaction of physical/cognitive development and external world.
- Cultural   – role of cultural (and social) factors in development of intelligence.
- Systems   – multiple, interacting intelligences rather than one 'best' approach.

Clearly these approaches, while distinct, may nevertheless be complementary, as reflected in the growing popularity of systems approaches to intelligence.

If some common factor is sought in these approaches it is the assumption that intellectual or cognitive ability varies across individuals in a way that may be measured and reflects the influence of other factors, whether these be genetic, developmental, cultural, etc. The most common area of debate is whether there exists a general factor (g) that underlies all intellectual functioning, or whether instead intelligence reflects a constellation of specific abilities (e.g. verbal, spatial) which are only loosely related.

Components of intelligence

There is still a great deal of interest in the search for a general factor of intelligence, this currently being regarded as the direct correlate of some underlying neural or physiological substrate of intelligence, for example speed (or accuracy) of neural transmission. The majority of psychometric tests of intelligence include several sub-scales (e.g. verbal intelligence). The fact that these sub-scales tend to be highly correlated is used to support the notion of some superordinate general factor, as is the fact that across diverse cultures there is always some semantic equivalent of dispositional adjectives such as 'bright', 'smart', and so on. Several distinctions have been postulated to clarify the structure of intelligence:

- *Fluid intelligence* is the aspect of intelligence which allows for the solution of novel problems and the use of creativity.
- *Crystallised intelligence*, in contrast, is the knowledge utilisation of specific, learned facts and the application of logical solutions to concrete problems.

Several investigators (most recently Eysenck) have suggested that intelligence is reflected at different levels:

- Biological   – that is, the neural substrate of intelligence.
- Behavioural   – the reflection of general intelligence in behaviour (e.g. exam success).
- Psychometric – as measured by intelligence tests.

The majority of psychometric tests of intelligence use factor analysis as a means of clustering test items into groups, which are suggested to reflect sub-scales of intelligence, or components of intelligence. The number of these varies greatly across tests. For example, the Stanford–Binet Intelligence Scale includes sub-scales of verbal reasoning, quantitative reasoning and visual reasoning, among others. The Wechsler Adult Intelligence Scale (WAIS), on the other hand, has only two distinct parts: a verbal intelligence scale and a performance intelligence scale. Separate scales for use with children also exist (e.g. Wechsler Intelligence Scale for Children; WISC).

Intelligence quotient (IQ)

Strictly, IQ is the mental age of a subject, divided by chronological age and multiplied by 100. This defines the mean intelligence within a given population as 100. Mental age is assessed by means of a standardised test. IQ was originally envisaged as a means of identifying intellectually retarded school children with a view to selection for special educational programmes. Recently, the emphasis on mental or intellectual age and chronological age has been reduced, largely because in adults such a concept is meaningless (intellectual ability does not continue to increase through the lifespan, while chronological age clearly does).

A more useful definition of IQ is the ratio between the score by an individual on a specific test and the norm for that individual's age group, multiplied by 100. This more general definition has supplanted the original definition (see above) of intelligence quotient.

The controversy associated with IQ tests has stemmed from the abuse that the concept has allowed: for example, to lend specious scientific credibility to racial prejudice. Nevertheless, interest in the area remains, and the value of tests of intellectual ability is clear as long as the limitations are well understood. Given that intelligence quotient is defined with reference to the norm within a given population, for example, it is meaningless to make comparisons across populations (e.g. across races). Given that the majority of tests have been designed to make comparisons with or predictions of academic performance it is unsurprising that there is a subsequent emphasis on verbal and mathematical reasoning. Ultimately, intelligence must be defined as that which intelligence tests measure, and attempts to reverse this (i.e. determine what intelligence is from what intelligence tests measure) may well prove to be circular and unfruitful.

Measurement of intelligence

How intelligence is assessed will have a very direct influence on what is in fact being assessed. For example, the use of verbal materials in the assessment of intelligence may severely hamper those who experience difficulty with such materials, such as those for whom the test is in a second language, children or the mentally retarded. This may unfairly represent these subjects as very low in intelligence, and consequently tests have been constructed which reduce such material to a minimum.

Measurement also depends on the assumptions made about the nature of intelligence (see above). The majority of intelligence tests rely on one of two theoretical frameworks:

- *Psychometric*: factor analysis of intelligence test items tends to reveal a number of specific factors (verbal, visual, etc.), which usually correlate (suggested by some to imply a general factor). Predictive power of tests that include several specific factors of intelligence tends to be no greater than general tests that include few factors. A major problem with this approach, then, is the lack of consensus on the number of factors that constitute intelligence.
- *Computational*: more recent information-processing approaches to intelligence suggest that the means by which problems are solved is more fundamental, and therefore more revealing, than the actual ability to solve specific problems (as in psychometric tests). For example, a specific individual may display poor recall of items from memory (required to solve a problem) or choose an inappropriate strategy for solving the problem.

Psychometric approaches, then, allow for rapid measurement of general aspects of intelligence, while computational approaches allow for a detailed, qualitative profile of intellectual function to be constructed. The two approaches may be seen as complementary. The quality of intellectual deficit may reveal specific neurological deficits, for example following brain injury, and is likely to be more revealing than a global, quantitative assessment of intelligence.

Computational models of intelligence propose five information-processing components:

- Metacomponents   – higher-order control, choice of strategy.
- Performance components   – execution of strategies.
- Acquisition components   – learning processes, acquisition of knowledge.
- Retention components   – memory processes, retrieval of knowledge.
- Transfer components   – transfer of knowledge from one situation to another.

Cultural influences

The role of intercultural and intracultural influences on intelligence has perhaps generated the greatest controversy, in particular the use of intelligence tests as justification for racial discrimination. This abuse of intelligence tests has greatly hindered progress in this area, and rests on a misapplication of such tests. Given that intelligence tests are designed for use within tightly defined populations, comparisons made across populations are meaningless, since the tests are only valid for within-population comparisons. Attempts to include culturally unbiased items within intelligence tests simply reflect an attempt to broaden the population that the test may be used on. Given that intelligence tests are defined by the mean score achieved within a population (100), any population that does not show such a mean (as well as a normal distribution) cannot meaningfully be assessed by that test.

This cultural bias is exemplified by studies that have constructed intelligence tests for use in other cultures (e.g. Native American), with mean scores within that population of 100, and then applied these within Western cultures. Western subjects have achieved correspondingly poor scores on such tests.

Apparent racial and cultural differences in intelligence test scores may in fact be a reflection of some third factor. For example, intelligence tests administered to immigrants to the United States appeared to show lower scores for those of South European origin when compared with the scores of those of North European origin. In fact, the strongest relationship was between intelligence test score and duration of stay in the United States, with scores rising over time, eventually reaching 'normal' levels after 15–20 years. This is not surprising given the large proportion of items on early tests that reflected aspects of crystallised intelligence (e.g. 'How many dimes are there in a dollar?').

Summary

- *Intelligence* is by no means the same as *IQ*. This is not a controversial statement, but rather emphasises that no single satisfactory definition of intelligence exists, while IQ may be regarded as self-defining, being at the very least that which IQ tests assess (although this is not particularly enlightening). Many of the controversies associated with IQ tests result from their inappropriate usage or an overinterpretation of results. When discussing intelligence it is important to be aware of different 'types' of intelligence: psychometric, computational, biological and others.
- A perennial question in this area is whether there exists a general ('*g*') factor of intelligence, from which more specific abilities derive, or whether intelligence simply consists of the interaction between independent intellectual abilities (so that there is greater choice as to which abilities should be included in any definition of intelligence). Note also the distinction between crystallised and fluid intelligence.
- Intelligence is traditionally measured by means of a questionnaire, sometimes including tasks which have to be performed. This *psychometric approach* has been challenged recently by *computational approaches* that suggest that the method used to solve a problem is more revealing than whether or not the problem is solved. Several factors influence intelligence test performance, and it is here that the interpretation of results should proceed with care. Talk of cultural influences is, to an extent, meaningless as tests are constructed to be used within tightly defined populations.

NEUROPSYCHOLOGICAL ASSESSMENT

Evaluations may take different forms:

- *Diagnostic assessments* focus on the normal and abnormal nature of overall functioning, and may include clinical interviews, mental state examinations and psychometric testing. They may be brief and focus on specific concerns, or be lengthy and comprehensive, depending on the specific issues being addressed.
- *Neuropsychological assessments* are more focused and typically lengthier, and are designed to test neuropsychological functioning by means of a

battery of tests that may take up to 8 hours to complete. The focus is on the process of neurological functioning and assessments of this type should not be confused with neurological tests (such as fMRI and CT scans) that focus on structure.

Neuropsychological assessment rests on certain assumptions, namely that:

- brain function is related to cognitive function;
- brain damage is related to cognitive deficit;
- cognitive deficit will be reflected in behaviour; and
- behavioural deficit will lead to social deficit.

This implies four levels of impaired function/deficit:

- Physical/physiological
- Cognitive
- Behavioural
- Social

Neuropsychological assessment is most valuable in cases of traumatic brain injury or in patients with impaired cognitive function as a result of organic disease. The primary purposes of such an assessment are the diagnosis of the patient condition and the analysis of progress (below). Such assessment procedures are also used in children to assess cognitive development and in patients with learning disabilities.

The components of any assessment may include some or all of:

- *Clinical interview*, which may be structured to a greater or lesser degree, where the emphasis is primarily on history gathering, focusing on the development of the individual and of the presenting problem.
- *Mental status examination*, usually conducted as part of the clinical interview, where thought processes, emotions and interpersonal qualities are assessed, usually relatively crudely and quickly to guide further assessment.
- *Objective personality* and *mood tests*, using validated psychometric instruments such as the Minnesota Multiphasic Personality Inventory and the Beck Depression Inventory, where population norms for comparison exist.
- *Projective personality tests*, better regarded as idiographic clinical tools rather than nomographic tests, including such tests as the Rorschach Inkblot Test and the Thematic Apperception Test.
- *Aptitude tests*, designed to assess cognitive and intellectual functioning, such as the Wechsler Adult Intelligence Scale and the Wechsler Intelligence Scale for Children, where poor performance on a single sub-scale may be informative of localised deficit.

Intelligence tests are commonly used to assess cognitive function, but a moderate score may reflect severe deficit in one area that is masked by good function in other aspects. As such, the quality of performance on such tests is often most revealing, and requires close inspection by the assessing individual given that, although distinct, performance on sub-scales of aptitude tests are typically highly correlated in normal individuals, so that localised deficit on a single sub-scale may reflect localised neuropsychological deficit.

A standard assessment of mental status or cognitive function will include several components:

- Immediate memory – similar to STM of psychologists, recall after several seconds.
- Short-term memory – *not* the STM of psychologists, memory over few minutes.
- Medium-term memory – memories for events over past week.
- Factual knowledge – news items, current events.
- Attention span – counting backwards in threes, etc.
- Orientation – in time and place.

Roth *et al.* (1990) suggest several purposes of functional assessment in order to:

- quantify patient function;
- describe the level of ability in self-care and mobility;
- monitor changes in status;
- guide management decisions;
- evaluate treatment efficacy;
- prevent additional disability;
- predict prognosis;
- plan placement;
- estimate care requirements; and
- determine compensation.

Clearly, the exact goal of assessment will vary widely across situations, and also as a function of who is carrying out the assessment.

Summary

- The four levels at which human behaviour may be understood (physical/physiological, cognitive, behavioural and social) may be applied to the study of impaired function, so that impairment at one level may be expected to have an impact on function at higher levels. One should be aware of the assumptions on which *neuropsychological assessment* rests.

- There are several components to any standard assessment: immediate memory; short-term memory (where the distinction between psychologists' STM and psychiatrists' STM is important); medium-term memory; factual knowledge; attention span; and orientation. It is often the quality, rather than the quantity, of impairment or performance that is most revealing about the nature of the subject's deficit.

PSYCHOLOGICAL ASSESSMENT INDIVIDUAL STATEMENT QUESTIONS

The following statements are either true or false:

1. In the Wechsler intelligence scales, 'hold' and 'don't hold' sub-tests refer to effects of normal ageing.
2. In the Wechsler intelligence scales, a low score on the coding sub-test can result from motor difficulties.
3. In the Wechsler intelligence scales, organic brain disease tends to depress performance scales scores more than verbal scales scores.
4. In the Wechsler intelligence scales, unexpectedly poor scores should be checked by re-testing within 2 weeks.
5. In the Wechsler intelligence scales, most normal individuals will have similar scores on all sub-tests.

6. In the construction of a psychometric rating scale, high measures of test–retest reliability may impair the detection of individual change.
7. In the construction of a psychometric rating scale, factor analysis of items provides a measure of concurrent validity.
8. In the construction of a psychometric rating scale, construct validity relates the scale to a heuristic theory.
9. In the construction of a psychometric rating scale, the type of population chosen for standardisation must be different from the population for which the scale is intended.
10. In the construction of a psychometric rating scale, internal consistency is indicated by assessing split-half reliability.

11. Sources of error in a self-administered questionnaire include response set.
12. Sources of error in a self-administered questionnaire include control tendency.
13. Sources of error in a self-administered questionnaire include social desirability.
14. Sources of error in a self-administered questionnaire include defensiveness.
15. Sources of error in a self-administered questionnaire include obsessionality.

16. The Wechsler scales for assessing intelligence are standardised on population norms.
17. The Wechsler scales for assessing intelligence use a ratio of mental age to chronological age to calculate IQ.
18. The Wechsler scales for assessing intelligence yield a full scale IQ by averaging performance and verbal scale scores.
19. The Wechsler scales for assessing intelligence in their revised form are culture-free.
20. The Wechsler scales for assessing intelligence can be administered by telephone.

21. Frequency ratings are likely to be used in the behavioural assessment of a problem.
22. Interviews are likely to be used in the behavioural assessment of a problem.
23. Baselining is likely to be used in the behavioural assessment of a problem.
24. Self-rating is likely to be used in the behavioural assessment of a problem.
25. IQ testing is likely to be used in the behavioural assessment of a problem.

26. Assessment of a patient with obsessive-compulsive disorder for behavioural psychotherapy is likely to focus on current symptoms.
27. Assessment of a patient with obsessive-compulsive disorder for behavioural psychotherapy is likely to involve measurement of a baseline.
28. Assessment of a patient with obsessive-compulsive disorder for behavioural psychotherapy is likely to involve mental state examination.
29. Assessment of a patient with obsessive-compulsive disorder for behavioural psychotherapy is likely to be completed in about 30 minutes.
30. Assessment of a patient with obsessive-compulsive disorder for behavioural psychotherapy is likely to involve consideration of target setting.

31. Functional assessment of a behavioural problem entails exploring antecedents to the behaviour.
32. Functional assessment of a behavioural problem entails exploring early life events.
33. Functional assessment of a behavioural problem entails exploring the part others play in reinforcement.
34. Functional assessment of a behavioural problem entails exploring the results of the behaviour.
35. Functional assessment of a behavioural problem entails the assessment taking about 30 minutes.

36. In behavioural assessment, baselining is important.
37. In behavioural assessment, rating scales are valuable.
38. In behavioural assessment, the focus is on present symptoms.
39. In behavioural assessment, attention is paid in good detail to reasons for the behaviour.
40. In behavioural assessment, a good therapeutic relationship with the therapist is vital.

41. Self-monitoring will form part of the behavioural analysis of a case of panic disorder.
42. Elucidation of cues will form part of the behavioural analysis of a case of panic disorder elucidation of cues.
43. Biofeedback will form part of the behavioural analysis of a case of panic disorder.
44. The role of family relationships will form part of the behavioural analysis of a case of panic disorder description.
45. The role of antecedent events will form part of the behavioural analysis of a case of panic disorder listing.

46. In testing disturbances on information processing, the Continuous Performance Test (CPT) involves the presentation of target stimuli among random stimuli on a computer screen.
47. In testing disturbances on information processing, short-term recall memory deficits occur in schizophrenia.
48. In testing disturbances on information processing, a pendulum can be used to test smooth eye pursuit movement.
49. In testing disturbances on information processing, there is no relationship between smooth eye pursuit movement dysfunction and schizophrenia.
50. In testing disturbances on information processing, the Wisconsin Card Sorting Test measures temporal lobe dysfunction.

51. In assessing personality, the Minnesota Multiphasic Personality Inventory has a schizophrenia scale.
52. In assessing personality, the California Personality Inventory was developed for a psychiatric population.
53. In assessing personality, the Thematic Apperception Test involves the presentation of ten stories.
54. In assessing personality, traits show considerable personal consistency over time.
55. In assessing personality, the Rorschach inkblot test is a projective technique.

56. Rating scales to measure locus of control were introduced by Rotter (1966).
57. Rating scales exist to measure the cognitive aspects of pain.
58. Rating scales can be used to assess psychotherapy outcome, but not psychotherapy process.
59. Rating scales such as the Life Events Scales (Paykel, 1971) rely on observer ratings of taped interviews about events.
60. Rating scales such as the Bulimic Investigatory Test (Henderson and Freeman, 1987) are designed to measure bulimic behaviour in inpatients.

61. Construct validity is evaluated by investigating what qualities a test measures.
62. Convergent validity is held to be established when measures that are predicted to be associated are found not to be related.
63. Divergent validity is where measures discriminate between other measures of related constructs.

64. Face validity can be determined by statistical methods.
65. Cross-validation may involve assessing criterion validity in different populations.

ANSWERS

1.	T	23.	T	45.	F
2.	F	24.	T	46.	T
3.	T	25.	F	47.	T
4.	F	26.	T	48.	T
5.	T	27.	T	49.	F
6.	T	28.	T	50.	F
7.	F	29.	F	51.	T
8.	F	30.	T	52.	F
9.	F	31.	T	53.	F
10.	T	32.	F	54.	T
11.	T	33.	T	55.	T
12.	F	34.	T	56.	T
13.	T	35.	F	57.	T
14.	F	36.	T	58.	F
15.	F	37.	T	59.	F
16.	T	38.	T	60.	F
17.	F	39.	F	61.	T
18.	F	40.	F	62.	F
19.	F	41.	T	63.	F
20.	F	42.	T	64.	F
21.	T	43.	F	65.	T
22.	T	44.	F		

2

Human development

---

5 Human development   119

5

Human development

Conceptual frameworks	119	Sexual development	156
Methodologies	126	Adolescence	159
Attachment theory	128	Adaptations in adult life	162
Family relationships	133	Pregnancy and childbirth	165
Temperament	138	Development of personal identity	167
Cognitive development	142	Ageing	170
Language development	145	Disability and pain	172
Social development	149	Death and dying	174
Moral development	152	Human development individual	176
Development of fears	154	statement questions	

CONCEPTUAL FRAMEWORKS

Nature and nurture

A great deal of research has focused on the question of whether specific abilities are inherited (nature) or learned (nurture). This approach, in its crudest sense, is invalid as very few abilities can be attributed to entirely genetic or environmental factors. Instead, the two should be regarded as interactive (see below). For example, even the physical development of the foetus, for example, may be affected by environmental factors (e.g. German measles), while the single gene disorder phenylketonuria can be entirely prevented if appropriate dietary treatment is given to the mother.

In most cases, genetic factors provide a set of parameters within which the infant can develop, with the exact nature of that development being influenced by the environment. These parameters are broadly similar across all infants, so that motor development proceeds in a uniform series of stages as the infant matures. The exact age at which a child begins to walk or speak is perhaps less important than the fact that this must be preceded by accomplishment of other tasks. That genetic factors set the range of development of a particular characteristic is evident in that, while humans vary greatly in height we would never expect to find an individual who was 3 metres tall, since there is an upper limit to height, even in an optimal environment. This may explain why racehorse breeding has failed to significantly increase the speed of racehorses over the past hundred years: previous breeding may have resulted in the upper limit being reached already.

The statistic used to calculate the relative contribution of genotype and environment to the observed phenotype, heritability, is also widely misunderstood. This is a population statistic that provides information on the proportion of *variability* in the observed phenotype that may be accounted for by variability in the genotype and variability in the environment. Therefore, the number of fingers on a hand, while genetically determined, is not highly heritable as any *variation* in this number is generally the result of environmental factors. Height, however, is highly heritable since most diets – even relatively poor ones – are sufficient to promote growth, so that variation in height is the result of genetic factors. This latter example also indicates that a heritability statistic for a given phenotype is specific to the time and population on which it was calculated: in populations where the diet is more variable, more of the variation in height in *that* population may be associated with this effect, so that the heritability coefficient will be different even if the underlying distribution of genes is the same.

Stage theories

Evidence from the development of linguistic and motor ability suggests that specific stages of development exist for different abilities. The assumption of stage theories is that these specific stages represent necessary conditions for the development of subsequent abilities. That is, infants learn to walk via a process of rolling over, crawling, etc., with walking representing a relatively late stage of development that cannot be reached until previous stages have been passed through. The order of these stages is invariant, with environmental factors influencing only the rate at which stages are completed. Piaget described his model of cognitive development in infants and genetic epistemology; meaning that the basic prerequisites for initiating development, such as crude motor skills, were inherited. When these prerequisites were enacted in a typical environment, the consequence would be feedback that would stimulate development (as opposed to maturation; see below). So, the infant's behaviour results in consequences that provide further information about the environment and the infant's relationship with it, which allows a greater understanding of that environment to develop. For example, the act of repeatedly banging objects against a hard surface provides information about which types of object are breakable and which are not.

Central to the concept of stage theories is the notion of specific periods (critical periods) that represent the transition from one stage to the next. Motor ability, for example, while developing at very different rates across individuals, may nevertheless be expected to be complete by the end of a specific critical period. There is clear evidence for the existence of critical periods in the physical development of infants and, to a lesser extent, also in cognitive development. In the latter case, a critical period represents the acquisition of the requisite cognitive skills to allow a qualitative change in subsequent cognition.

While the suggestion of qualitatively distinct stages of development is well supported for physical development, the use of this theoretical framework in understanding psychological development is less well supported. A common criticism of such approaches (e.g. Piaget; see below) is that the responses of infants and children are highly susceptible to experimenter influences or the characteristics of the experiment itself.

Maturational tasks

The critical periods described above are brought about by the performance of specific tasks. For example, standing unaided precedes walking, and initial walking is clumsy, gradually being refined. Maturational tasks are suggested to be necessary behaviours that allow more complex behaviours to develop. For example, standing is necessary for walking to take place, and as such the infant must become accomplished at this before attempting to walk any distance. These tasks, then, drive progress through specific stages and critical periods in development.

The concept of *maturation* is closely allied to the discussion of the relative influences of nature and nurture (see above), or genes and environment. The behaviours that allow maturational tasks to be completed are largely genetically determined, so that as time progresses these behaviours develop accordingly. The practice that the infant gets, however, is environmentally determined, so that there are cultural differences in motor development, for example, on the basis of the encouragement given to infants to perform these maturational tasks. Again, the applicability of this framework to psychological development is not universally accepted. It is also important to distinguish between simple maturation, which is pure biological unfolding driven primarily by genetic factors given basic environmental input such as diet, and development, which is the sequence of changes over the lifespan of the individual and results from the interaction between behaviours (some a consequence of maturation) and the environment.

Maturity

Maturity is a necessarily broad term, and as such is difficult to define. Most simply, it may be regarded as the culmination (i.e. end-point) of the maturational (and developmental) processes described above. Maturity may also, however, be considered as its components, so that we may refer to sexual maturity as distinct from, say, cognitive or intellectual maturity. While physical maturity (e.g. sexual) may be quite tightly defined, maturity of psychological characteristics is more problematic and subjective. Subsequent discussion of cognitive and moral development will note that a large proportion of the adult population never reaches the final stages of such development (cf. Piaget, 1929; Kohlberg, 1981), and as such may be said to not reach maturity, although clearly only in a specific and technical sense.

Gene–environment interactions

The broad implications of interactions between genetic and environmental influences have been described above. More specific implications have contributed to the debate concerning the nature and development of intelligence and personality, both of which have been claimed to be up to 80% heritable (see above), although most estimates range from 50 to 60%. While twin studies and other methods have certainly suggested a genetic component to intellectual ability, the interpretation of these results is problematic given the highly interactive nature of the factors in question, and the complex nature of intelligence itself.

Early, simple additive models of intelligence suggested that genotype and environment both contributed independently to the phenotypic expression of intelligence, so that the relative contribution could be determined by certain experimental means (e.g. the comparison of identical twins raised apart, or the comparison of monozygotic versus dizygotic twins). Notwithstanding the methodological weaknesses of many of these studies (and a few celebrated scientific frauds), the model of genetic influence guiding this research is potentially inappropriate. The following model of genotype–phenotype interaction, proposed by Scarr and McCartney (1983), highlights this.

While the genotype and environment of an individual will doubtless influence the phenotype of that individual, several other influences also exist. Most importantly, the phenotype of the individual will influence the environment, so that physically short individuals will be less likely to find themselves playing basketball. In this sense, it would be possible to find a genetic component for basketball-playing, but this would not be interpreted as a gene 'for' basketball (whereas comparable findings in intelligence are so interpreted). Rather, the combined influence of a number of genes related to physical development, when expressed in a given context (i.e. a population where basketball was played), would influence the likelihood of an individual playing basketball. The various influences in this interactive model include:

- Child's genotype on child's phenotype
- Child's environment on child's phenotype
- Child's phenotype on child's environment
- Parents' genotype on child's genotype
- Parents' genotype on child's environment
- External influences on child's environment

The influence of the parents' genotype on the child's environment may also, because of the obvious genetic relationship between parents and child, appear as a genetic influence, rather than an environmental one. Finally, because of certain cultural norms certain physical characteristics will result in the individual being treated in a certain way. Attractive children, for example, are likely to receive more stimulation in infancy, which may result in faster or improved cognitive development. This may appear as a genetic influence, even though the gene found is 'for' physical attractiveness that, in a specific culture, results in certain treatment that may facilitate intellectual development, so that the genetic influence is mediated by a culturally-determined environmental influence. In this case it would be more proper to call the environmental mediating variable causal, rather than the genetic variable.

Early and late adversities

The interactive model of physical and psychological development has application to the understanding of the aetiology of psychiatric disorders. In particular, various affective disorders are known to depend on both inherited factors (e.g. neurotransmitter activity) and childhood environment (e.g. parenting style). Cognitive models of depression, for example, suggest a role for self-schema, which represent models of the self and the relationship of the self to others, as a potential vulnerability factor (or protective factor). These self-schema develop gradually in early life and will depend on personal experiences. This suggests that once such schemas have become established they will become self-sustaining, so that early experiences will be more important than late experiences. Nevertheless, depression is commonly associated with a major, negative life event, so that a role exists for later experiences, although this is a very different role. Of note are the following:

- Genetic factors   – e.g. dopamine in schizophrenia.
- Psychological factors   – e.g. self-schema in depression.
- Environmental factors   – e.g. life events, major stressors.

Other distortions in cognitive and emotional development may be of relevance in understanding personality disorders, in particular problems of social skills and self-concept. Generally, events in early life will influence the development of risk factors such as self-concept, social skills, etc., while later events will act as causal factors given the existence of such risk or protective factors. It is important not to focus primarily on the existence of risk factors. It can be as informative to ask why some individuals do *not* develop, for example, an affective disorder following a significant negative life event. This accounts for the apparent resilience found in some individuals, where appropriate early experiences and subsequent emotional and cognitive development may act as protective factors.

Psychoanalytic theories

General psychoanalytic theories suggest that development represents a process whereby instinctive behaviours are gradually reformed so as to become socially acceptable, requiring in many instances the repression of such behaviour (e.g. Freud). Note that such theories suggest that cognitive, emotional and especially social development is a largely passive process, with the infant playing little part in his or her own development.

Social learning theory

This is a very general model of·learning that is predicated on the ability of individuals to learn from the observation of others. In infants, sexual identity, for example, is suggested to be learned by a process of modelling the appropriate parent's behaviour. This process of modelling may be guided (for example, by the parent demonstrating a behaviour) or automatic (in which case it is not necessarily a conscious process). While social learning theory may be applied at all developmental stages including adulthood, it is of most relevance in early life when the child is far more susceptible to modelling processes, and learning in general.

Piaget

The genetic epistemology of Piaget is discussed in more detail in other sections. Based almost entirely on the observations of his own children, Piaget developed a detailed stage theory of cognitive development, with a strong emphasis on the interaction between biological predispositions and environmental influence. Specifically, infants are born with a set of instinctive behaviours that lead to the gradual development of knowledge about the world and others as a result of the consequences of these behaviours. Of note are the following:

- Schemas — models of how the world operates (physical and social).
- Assimilation — attempt to understand novel experience with reference to schemas.
- Accommodation — modification of schemas to incorporate novel experience.

The most important (and widely accepted) contribution of Piaget is his description of the infant as actively contributing to his/her own development as a result of his interaction with the physical and social worlds, driven by simple, inherited behavioural predispositions.

Summary

- Understanding human development often employs stage theories, which suggest that development (cognitive, emotional, social, etc.) occurs in distinct stages, with the completion of a stage being a necessary condition for advancement to the next stage. The most well-known stage theory is *Piaget's theory* of cognitive development. A related concept is that of *maturational tasks*, which are specific tasks that must be performed in order for a stage to be completed. For example, understanding that objects continue to exist when unseen is necessary in order for more complex understanding of the relationship between the individual and external objects to be possible.
- Debate over the relative influence of genetic and environmental factors on *phenotypic expression* is popularly referred to as the nature–nurture debate. A reasonable position from which to begin is to accept that most human characteristics may vary within limits defined largely by the genotype, while much variation within these limits may be accounted for by environmental factors. More importantly, genetic and environmental factors are not simply additive and may interact in complex ways. Piaget's theory of cognitive development, suggests that specific behaviours are innate (i.e. genetically determined), but the expression of these in a social context results in learning and cognitive development. The relative influence of genetic and environmental factors varies with age, which provides an indication of 'risk periods' when the child may be vulnerable to the impact of early adversities.

- One should be aware of several key theoretical frameworks, in particular Piaget's theory of cognitive and intellectual development, Kohlberg's theory of moral development (another stage theory), the general principles of *psychoanalytic theory*, where development is seen as a largely passive process, and *social learning theory*. The latter represents an attempt to integrate several theoretical positions and emphasises that development takes place in a social context where appropriate behaviour is rewarded and inappropriate behaviour punished.

METHODOLOGIES

Cross-sectional

Cross-sectional methodologies, used in studies of human development, employ large groups of subjects who are studied at one time only. This presents a snapshot of the chosen population at a certain stage of development, but provides little or no information about the underlying developmental processes that have resulted in current status. This may be achieved by the collection of retrospective data, usually by self-report, but this obviously is potentially flawed and of questionable reliability and validity. Nevertheless, it is an efficient way to collect large amounts of data that may potentially allow the discrimination between groups that may subsequently be related to antecedent, developmental events.

Cohort

In cohort studies, subjects are chosen on the basis of one or more unifying characteristics. For example, longitudinal studies of the genetic and environmental risk factors for schizophrenia commonly investigate the children of schizophrenic parents, as the incidence of schizophrenia in such subjects is far higher than in the normal population. This is convenient, but presents a problem concerning the generalisability of results obtained from such studies. Longitudinal studies also require substantial resources to sustain them over a sufficiently lengthy period to allow the impact of the factors of interest to be realised.

Individual

Longitudinal studies of an individual allow the entire resources of a research project to be dedicated to the analysis of a single individual, so that far more detail is possible. Such idiographic methods, however, raise questions about the generalisability of results. Furthermore, this approach is not practical if the risk factors for a relatively uncommon condition are sought, as the likelihood of the individual developing the condition will be low. Cohort studies may allow for the identification of general risk characteristics such that individual studies then become practical. For example, the incidence of schizophrenia in the children of schizophrenic parents is still only c.10%, which is too low for individual studies to be practical.

Identification and evaluation of influences

There is substantial current interest in the relative influence of genetic and environmental factors on development (see pp. 119–120). Methodologies for investigating this rely on comparison being made along certain phenotypic dimensions between individuals of varying genetic similarity. For example, identical (monozygotic or MZ) twins are genetically identical, while normal siblings (dizygotic or DZ) twins only share one half of their genes. As such, if a psychological characteristic is more strongly correlated in MZ twins compared to DZ twins, this suggests a genetic influence. Note that this methodology relies on a simple additive model of genetic and environmental influence that is probably inadequate (see earlier discussion, p. 122). Several varying degrees of genetic and environmental similarity are possible:

- MZ twins reared together.
- MZ twins reared apart.
- DZ twins reared together.
- Siblings reared together.
- Siblings reared apart.
- Cousins.
- Adopted children reared together.

Other combinations are possible, but this demonstrates the variety of comparisons that may be made. On a variety of phenotypic characteristics (e.g. personality and other psychological dimensions) the degree of similarity between individuals increases with genetic similarity (and also with environmental similarity). The interpretation of such results, however, is highly problematic, and it is becoming increasingly clear that an accurate characterisation and reliable measurement of the phenotypic characteristic of interest is of primary importance.

Summary

- Three main methodologies have been employed in the investigation of human development: cross-sectional designs, cohort designs and longitudinal studies of individuals. The first method studies large groups at a single point in time, while the second selects a group on the basis of a common characteristic (e.g. risk for schizophrenia). The third approach devotes large resources to the detailed study of an individual and is therefore quite distinct from the first two approaches.
- Studies which investigate the relative influence of genetic and environmental factors on a phenotypic characteristic make comparisons between individuals with varying degrees of genetic and environmental similarity, on the assumption that if an effect is due to, say, genetic influence then the greater the degree of similarity the greater the degree of similarity in the dependent characteristic. One should be aware of the difficulties associated with interpreting results from such studies.

ATTACHMENT THEORY

Attachment theory describes the behaviours of infants (in primates generally) towards adults, and the progression of these behaviours as they gradually become focused on one (or, occasionally, more than one) attachment figure. The desire for proximity and affection displayed by such infants is in fact natural and genetically determined behaviour that is a necessary precursor to the psychological, emotional and social development of the infant. The first attachment figure (usually the mother, but not necessarily so) serves as the paradigm for the development of future relationships. Note that:

- Attachment behaviour — the behaviours displayed by young infants towards mother, etc.
- Attachment figure — focus of attachment behaviours, e.g. receptive to care from mother.

In the first few (c. 6) months, the infant does not display selectivity in the direction of behaviour, but after this period attachment behaviours specifically directed towards an attachment figure (commonly, although probably not necessarily, the mother) become apparent. This represents the formation of an attachment with that figure, and interestingly does not depend primarily on feeding but instead on affection, caring, and so on. Survival behaviours (i.e. seeking food, etc.) appear to be somewhat dissociated from attachment behaviours (i.e. seeking love, affection, etc.) and serve a more social purpose. This has been shown in animal studies, where rhesus monkeys separated from their mother will spend the majority of time clinging to a wool doll rather than a wire doll, even when it is the latter which provides food. Presumably, the triggers for attachment behaviour are not related to feeding, and are instead related to proximity, nurturance and so on that are cued by other stimuli (such as the physical characteristics of the mother):

- Evolutionary basis – infant's best hope for survival lies in proximity to caretaker.
- Early weeks   – infant is predisposed to achieve closeness.
- 3rd month   – attachment remains indiscriminate and transient.
- 6th month   – (usually) single attachment figure established.
- 12th month   – fear of strangers, attachment maintained over distance.
- 24th month   – attachment figure (usually mother) of primary importance.
- 36th month   – substitute attachment figures accepted in absence of primary.
- Adulthood   – early attachment behaviour related to emotional development.

It has been widely suggested that the initial attachment forms a template for the development of subsequent social and emotional relationships, so that early behaviour may be predictive of later social behaviour. Different patterns of secure and insecure attachment behaviour will be discussed below.

Emotional development

The attachment behaviours displayed by an infant in early life appear to be highly correlated with subsequent development and behaviour. Secure attachment (see below) is related in later childhood with initiative taking, social competence and the ability to form friendships. Insecure attachment, on the other hand, is related to subsequent social withdrawal and difficulty in forming friendships. While not rigid, attachment behaviour seems to be relatively stable, once established, over the lifespan.

Affect regulation

Insecure attachment behaviours include the inability to express affection in a comfortable way with the attachment figure, either by being excessively dependent and at the same time irritated by the attachment figure, or by displaying avoidant behaviour (see p. 131 for more detail). The extent to which this is related to affect regulation in adult life is unclear, but given that attachment behaviours appear to be somewhat related to adult behaviour it is plausible that some relationship may exist. Generally, insecure attachments have been found to be related to emotional disturbance in adolescence and adulthood, although the strength of the relationship is only modest.

Relationships

The primary attachment figure serves as the paradigm for the development of subsequent relationships, including casual and close friendships as well as romantic relationships. There is some evidence that patterns of adult romantic relationships follow a similar pattern to attachment behaviours, with the proportion of adults describing themselves as within each category roughly corresponding to the proportions found in infant attachment styles. Retrospective questionnaires suggest that these styles of romantic affection are related to the perceived/remembered behaviour of the mother towards the individual, although there is a danger of circularity in this argument.

Secure attachment

Infants who display secure attachment behaviour use the attachment figure as a base from which to explore, occasionally returning to seek affection. Separation from the attachment figure (mother) induces anxiety and distress and interaction is sought on her return, although this may be brief. Anxiety subsequently reduces and exploration resumes. These behaviours are strongest/most evident during the first 36 months, after which separation anxiety gradually reduces and attachment substitutes may be accepted.

Secure attachment behaviour is related to:

- Child temperament (see discussion, p. 140).
- Child-focused caring/nurturing behaviour from the attachment figure.
- Encouragement for the child to explore independently from the attachment figure.
- Provision of a secure base by the attachment figure.

Insecure attachment

Insecure attachment behaviours comprise two distinct categories:

- *Insecure-avoidant behaviours* are characterised by muted distress in the absence of the attachment figure, and a minimal response on her/his return. What may appear to be secure, independent attachment behaviour may in fact be insecure-avoidant behaviour, and making the distinction may be difficult. The clearest difference lies in the fact that securely attached children still display closeness to the mother at times, balancing a desire for affection with independence, while insecure-avoidant children almost exclusively seek distance and self-sufficiency at the expense of closeness to the mother.

- *Insecure-ambivalent behaviours*, on the other hand, represent the least common attachment style, and children with such an attachment style display a curious mixture of excessively dependent behaviour towards the attachment figure allied with a lack of obvious affection. Separation results in excessive distress in the child but, on the return of the attachment figure, the child will then resist reunion and physical contact. Distress continues for some time after the return of the attachment figure.

There is some evidence for a relationship between insecure attachment styles and future antisocial behaviour and affective disorders. If such attachment behaviours are identified in early life, this may be countered by teaching parenting skills to the parents of the child, specifically to be more caring towards the child. Note, however, that it is far too simplistic to attribute attachment behaviours to the parenting style of the parents (see discussion of temperament, p. 138).

Early separation

Given the modest relationship between the development of secure attachments and subsequent behaviour in adolescence and adulthood, it may be expected that separation from initial attachment figures will be related to subsequent behavioural problems. This is related to the age at which such separation takes place. For example, selective attachments do not begin to form until the sixth month, so that separation before this time may be expected to have relatively little effect, allowing the formation of attachment behaviours towards the adoptive care-giver. There is evidence to support this. Similarly, after the first few years of life the child will have developed a pattern of attachment behaviour, and therefore a model or template of relationships, so that separation will not result in excessive disturbance to the child as it will be able to accept the adoptive care-giver as a substitute attachment figure.

The critical period, therefore, appears to be between the 6th and 36th months, when the greatest changes occur in the pattern of attachment behaviours and the understanding of relationship formation. Separation during this period is likely to have the greatest impact on the child's behaviour (see below), as it will disrupt the formation of normal attachment behaviour.

Failure to develop selective attachments

Autistic children are characterised by an unwillingness to seek physical contact with parents, being satisfied by their own company. This becomes most apparent between the 12th and 36th months, when normal, selective attachments would otherwise typically form. Clearly this is highly correlated with similar behaviour in adult life and appears to be largely the result of physical and genetic factors, rather than social or developmental processes.

The failure to develop selective attachments in autistic children as a result of internal factors should be distinguished from a breakdown of the normal attachment process because of external factors, i.e. the environment or the behaviour of potential attachment figures such as the parents. In this case, the lack of an obvious, single provider of care and affection results in incomplete development of attachment behaviours, so that strangers and parents are treated similarly, without any apparent stranger anxiety. At the same time, the behaviour towards such figures is superficial and any affection easily terminated, so that separation anxiety also does not occur. It is for this reason that early separation in the critical period (see above) is most detrimental to the child, in particular if the child is not placed in a caring adoptive or foster home.

Maternal bonding

The anxiety which results from separation of the child from the attachment figure is a necessary part of the development of secure attachments, since it is the return of the attachment figure which gives the child confidence in the attachment figure. This, in turn, gives the child confidence in relationships, understanding that they persist over time and distance. Note that the term 'maternal bonding' is potentially inappropriate in that, although usual in most Western cultures, it is not necessary that the primary attachment figure be the mother.

Summary

- *Attachment theory* is a framework for understanding the behaviour of infant primates whereby proximity and affection are sought (attachment behaviours) and appear to act as primary drives, in a similar way to hunger and thirst. An attachment relationship develops between the infant and the provider of such care (the *attachment figure*). This relationship is posited to serve as the prototype for the development of subsequent relationships of all kinds. Attempts have been made, with varying success, to relate infant attachment behaviour to adolescent and adult friendships and romantic relationships. Selective attachments usually do not form before the 6th month.
- Attachment to an attachment figure may be either secure or insecure, with the latter being further subdivided into avoidant and ambivalent. *Secure attachment* represents a relationship where the attachment figure is used as a base for independent exploration, and while separation from the attachment figure results in distress this quickly subsides on reunion. *Insecure-avoidant attachment* is characterised by a relative lack of distress on separation and a general tendency for affection to be muted. Apparent security masks an unwillingness to display closeness. *Insecure-ambivalent behaviour*, finally, represents excessive dependence allied with an unwillingness to display affection towards the attachment figure. There is some evidence for a relationship between attachment style (which may be evident as early as the 6th month) and subsequent antisocial behaviour and affective disturbance.
- The development of attachment behaviours, selective attachments and so on takes place largely during a period between the 6th and 36th months. It is important to realise the implications this has for separation of the child from the primary attachment figure (i.e. usually the mother), with this critical period being associated with the greatest impact on the child's behaviour if separation occurs.
- A failure to develop selective factors may be the result of internal factors (e.g. autism) or external factors (e.g. disturbed family function). The latter situation may also be related to early separation of the child from the primary attachment figure during the critical period (i.e. the first three years of life).

FAMILY RELATIONSHIPS

Parenting practice and parental attitudes

The behaviour of individuals towards their offspring, dedicated to their care, nurturance, etc. is of primary importance in determining attachment behaviours in infants, with these factors further interacting with temperamental features of the infant (see below).

Parenting style is commonly characterised along two (self-explanatory) dimensions:

- Restrictive–permissive.
- Loving–hostile.

Alternatively, three categories of parenting style have been suggested:

- Permissive   − warm and caring, while accepting unorthodox behaviour.
- Authoritarian-restrictive − less emotionally close and highly controlling.
- Authoritative   − enforce rules, demand achievement, yet warm and loving.

The development of the child clearly depends greatly on the parenting style adopted by the child's parents. For example, authoritarian-restrictive parents tend to have highly submissive children, while authoritative parents tend to have independent children (largely as a result of the emphasis placed on expressiveness within set boundaries).

The behaviour of the parents is most important in the early development of the child, and this establishes a pattern of behaviour in the child that is sustained over time. In particular, the *consistency* of the parents' behaviour towards the child, for example with reference to the rewards and punishments consequent on certain behaviour, is a strong predictor of subsequent emotional and social behaviour in the child. Inconsistent parenting behaviour, presumably because it inhibits the development of clear social schema to guide behaviour, is associated with negative outcomes along these dimensions.

The extent to which specific attitudes of parents is mirrored in subsequent attitudes in their children is debatable: while there is certainly a relationship, there are also numerous examples of children adopting opposing attitudes and beliefs − in particular during adolescence. It is likely that parental behaviour that engenders independence in the child will result in less similarity of attitudes.

Distorted family function

There are a variety of ways in which normal family function may be distorted, some of which are discussed below. Such (dysfunctional) families are highly varied in the nature and extent of distorted function, so that care should be taken in making comparisons. Certainly there is no such thing as a typical dysfunctional family.

Distorted patterns of communication are often at the core of dysfunctional families, where complimentary or neutral remarks may be interpreted in a negative way. Such discord may be the consequence of misinterpretation or result of the way in which neutral comments are delivered (for example, in a sarcastic tone). This situation is frequently self-defeating as individuals attempt to exert their influence in response to perceived snubs or insults by reacting in a similar way. Conversely, behaviour that would be useful in reducing discord is rarely used (e.g. apology), and is typically seen by those involved as admissive of defeat.

Overprotection may be the result of enmeshment within a family (see below), in which case it is broadly applicable to all members of the family unit. It may also occur in specific cases; the central feature of overprotection is an unwillingness to allow a member of the family group to display any individuality, especially outside of the family group. The characteristic feature of such family behaviour is an apparent excess of closeness that is at the same time selfishly motivated.

Rejection may be a specific effect, where a mother, say, rejects closeness with her child, or a more general, family effect. In this latter case the family does not have a strong sense of collective identity, with individuals only showing weak attachment relationships to other members, often forming stronger attachments outside the family group. A sense of isolation and loneliness commonly results.

Enmeshment refers to families where individual identity and individuality is lost to family status and role, in direct contrast to rejection (see above). A high degree of homogeneity, especially of opinions and beliefs, results in little input in discussions regarding the family. Family structure is very tightly defined and any individual family member attempting to display some degree of independence is likely to have such behaviour suppressed.

Bereavement

Generally, 'bereavement' is used to describe the death of a loved one or relative, although it is sometimes used more generally (and metaphorically) to indicate loss of any kind (e.g. moving schools, leaving home, etc.). This latter use is based on some evidence that the reaction to loss of any kind follows a similar pattern, although the intensity of these reactions will vary. Typical reactions to bereavement (i.e. loss) include:

- Disbelief/denial.
- Emotional blunting/numbness.
- Excessive rumination over the lost object or individual.

Clearly, considerable adjustment is required in any case of bereavement, and the effect on a child is likely to be great. Behavioural problems are associated with the loss of a parent in children, and there is some evidence that this is related to poor adjustment in the surviving parent. It is difficult to establish the exact pattern of causation here. The subsequent development of the child is likely to be influenced most by the subsequent behaviour of the surviving parent (e.g. a change of parenting style, a relative neglect due to increased time demands, etc.), rather than loss of a parent *per se*.

Divorce

The effects of divorce on the development of the child are difficult to delineate, as parents who divorce have generally been in conflict for some time before the divorce, which will be of obvious relevance. In general, in the first year following a divorce:

- the parents of the child become more permissive/less controlling; and
- communication between parents and child deteriorates.

This behaviour is common to both the parent without the child and the parent who cares for the child. Usually, this change in parenting style resolves after the first year following the divorce. The effects of the divorce on the child depends on:

- the age of the child;
- the degree of hostility resulting from the divorce;
- the use of the child by the conflicting parents to achieve their own aims; and
- adjustment of the parent who remains caring for the child (see above).

In almost all cases there is a degree of distress in the child, allied to feelings of responsibility or guilt and consequent depression or hostility. In most cases, however, this resolves relatively quickly (i.e. after the first year), provided that the parent they remain with also adjusts over this time.

Intrafamilial abuse

Abuse of children is most dangerous in the early years of life (i.e. <4th year), not least because this is when the child is physically most vulnerable. This is also the time, however, when the antecedents of subsequent self-esteem and self-image are developing. Immediate effects of intrafamilial abuse (either physical or sexual) include:

- Sleep disturbance.
- Eating disturbance.
- Depression.
- Phobias/anxiety.
- Behavioural problems.
- Social problems.

The longer-term effects of abuse are more difficult to delineate, but there is some evidence that initial consequences (see above) may persist for several years if abuse continues. In particular, the following problems appear to persist:

- Depression (especially in sexual abuse).
- Self-harm/self-abuse.
- Low self-esteem.
- Impaired relationship formation.

These effects are greatest if the abuse comes from within the family group (which is the most common source), if the abuse is sustained over a substantial period, and if the abused is not believed when help is sought.

Non-orthodox family structures

The most common non-orthodox family structure is the single-parent family, a situation that has increased greatly in prevalence in recent years. This may be the result of bereavement (although this is rare), divorce (which is common) or single motherhood (which is also common and is increasing). The consequences of bereavement and divorce have already been discussed (see above). The consequences of living with only a mother (i.e. single-mother families) have also been investigated, since this is by far the most typical single-parent situation:

- *Self-identity*: boys, in particular, may have problems achieving a clear sexual identity if the father is absent in early life.
- *Gratification*: boys, again, are most affected and appear to show impaired ability to delay gratification and control impulses.
- *Social skills*: interaction with the opposite sex, in particular in girls, appears to be impaired.

There is also some evidence that the relative difficulty in forming relationships with the opposite sex found in the children of single mothers persist into adulthood, although the effect is a weak one. Moreover, the potential confound of differences in parenting behaviour existing in single-parent families is difficult to control for in studies that consider the impact of single-parent families on children, so that it is difficult to conclude that behavioural and psychological correlates of a single-parent upbringing are a consequence of the fact that only one parent was present.

Similar consequences for the development of the child have been found in other, very rare family structures (e.g. raised by grandparents).

While the extended family structure found in some cultures and ethnic groups should not be regarded as unorthodox, it is not the common structure in Western cultures. In general, children raised in such families tend to develop high levels of self-esteem and the family structure seems to represent a protective factor (i.e. by providing high levels of social support, etc.).

Summary

- Parenting style has been suggested to be a major determinant of child behaviour. The behaviour of the parents may be described as either *dimensional* (e.g. restrictive–permissive/loving–hostile) or *categorical* (e.g. permissive, restrictive, authoritative). There is evidence that parenting style does correlate with the behaviour of the child. For example, restrictive parents tend to have submissive children. This relationship is, of course, statistical, so that it is difficult to predict with any accuracy behaviour in the child from the behaviour of the parents in specific cases.
- It is important to understand that the impact of *bereavement* and *divorce* on family function, in particular children's behaviour, may be regarded under the more general term of loss. That is, there are certain similarities between bereavement and divorce, although clearly there also will be unique characteristics of each. Distress following loss of any kind is normal and should only be regarded as a problem if it becomes chronic in nature and extends beyond the normal time for adaptation and coping to take place.
- One should be aware of the specific terms used to describe different features of distorted family function, such as *overprotection*, *rejection* and *enmeshment*. While there is no such thing as a typical dysfunctional family, and the causes of dysfunction may vary widely, certain characteristics appear repeatedly (e.g. distorted or impoverished communication between family members).

TEMPERAMENT

Temperament and child–parent relationships

Infants, including newborns, display noticeable variation in behaviour from the moment of birth, to the extent that different infants may be regarded as possessing different personalities. Given that these differences are noticeable very soon after birth, it is plausible to suggest that some proportion of the variance in temperament (and, subsequently, personality in later life) is genetically determined. For example, one infant may be far more active than another, whereas others may vary in the ease with which they begin crying. Some enjoy physical contact far more than others. These differences will all influence the behaviour directed towards the infant, in particular by the parents. Therefore, interactions between infants and parents are a function of the child's temperament and behaviour and the parents' behaviour. On the assumption that development is driven by the interaction between innate behaviours and the changes in the environment (e.g. parents' behaviour) that these elicit, these differences in temperament may be an important factor in determining development.

Origins, typologies and stability of temperament

A 1950s study of temperament in children (carried out in the United States) interviewed mothers and assessed the behaviour of children of these along nine dimensions, identifying three types of temperament in the group studied:

- *Easy children* (c. 40%) were regular in sleeping and eating patterns, did not show great emotional lability, were playful and affectionate, and adapted readily and quickly to novel situations.
- *Slow-to-warm-up children* (c. 15%) differed in being less active overall and far slower at adapting to new situations, to the extent that novel situations were initially treated with suspicion/withdrawal.
- *Difficult children* (c. 10%) displayed little regularity in sleeping and eating patterns, were highly irritable and emotionally labile, and responded negatively to novel situations.

Note that this typology only accounts for c. 65% of children in the study, with the remaining one-third not being classified as clearly belonging to any of the categories. Follow-up of the majority of the sample provides some evidence for stability of temperament over time, although there are criticisms of the original interpretation of the data from the interviews conducted. Nevertheless, children classified as difficult are more likely to display school problems, while the correlation between behaviour and childhood temperament extends to adulthood. These correlations, while being significant, remained weak (c. 0.3).

The important assumption of studies of temperament is that the social and emotional development of the child is not simply the result of the behaviour of others (specifically, the parents). Instead, the child interacts with the world and others, modifying behaviour directed towards the child accordingly. This has implications for studies that attempt to determine the genetic components of personality and intelligence (see earlier discussion, p. 127), so that an apparent genetic effect may be the consequence of initial differences in, say, level of activity (i.e. active children are more likely to receive stimulation from others).

If it is assumed that the temperament of the child will interact with the behaviour of those caring for him or her, the 'goodness of fit' of the child's environment must be taken into account. That is, if a child displays a difficult temperament in early life, this may elicit highly negative responses from the parents. Alternatively, the parents may regard this as a positive challenge and display great patience with the child. The latter case is more likely to result in healthy development of the child.

Temperament and personality

It is a central question of developmental psychology whether the personality of older children and adults may be predicted from the behaviour and temperament of the young child. That is, to what extent is temperament reliable and persistent over time? Perhaps surprisingly, any continuity that does exist appears to be weak, presumably because of the strong environmental and societal influences on the development of personality. There is some evidence that the temperament of very young children is related to subsequent attachment behaviour (over a relatively short time span):

- Easy   – secure attachment.
- Slow-to-warm-up   – anxious avoidant attachment.
- Difficult   – anxious ambivalent attachment.

Attachment behaviour, in turn, has been shown to be weakly related to adult behaviour. The greater the temporal distance between temperament and current behaviour, however, the weaker the relationship.

Other dimensions of personality, however, have been more fruitful in providing insights into the interactions between genetic and environmental determinants. Extraversion–introversion, as a dimension of personality, appears to be in part genetically determined (by comparison of individual with varying genetic and environmental similarity), although it is unclear to what extent this is related to the current discussion of temperament and attachment.

While it is intuitively appealing that temperament is consistent over time, any consistency found between early temperament and subsequent behaviour is only evident for the first 5 years. Any consistency of behaviour beyond this appears to be primarily the result of parent–child interactions and the parenting style adopted by the family.

Vulnerability and resilience

Psychosocial adversity and life events are known to be related to mental illness, for example depression. The extent to which specific life events, for example, influence any individual varies greatly, so that it is important to talk of the degree of vulnerability and resilience an individual displays. While this is important in adult life, being described in terms of coping skills, etc., it is also of relevance in the understanding of children's mental health. There are a number of risk factors in childhood which have been suggested to be related to adult mental health:

- Family discord.
- Intrafamilial abuse.
- Early bereavement (especially mother/primary attachment figure).

However, it is unlikely that any strong link between these factors and adult mental health will ever be identified, as certain individuals display great resilience to such adversity. For example, children who display secure attachment behaviour are likely to be able to form replacement attachments if the mother is lost (depending on the age at which the loss occurs), resulting in a degree of resilience. It is entirely possible that early stress may result in resilience to subsequent stress in later life in some individuals and an increased vulnerability in others. The impact of early stress and adverse experiences will depend on temperamental factors and the emotional development of the child at the time of the stressful experience. Difficult and slow-to-warm-up temperamental types have been suggested as risk factors for subsequent behavioural difficulties (see above).

Summary

- In a similar way to the typology of attachment behaviour used to describe young infants, there have been attempts to categorise the behaviour of children. Three categories of temperament have been suggested: *easy*, *slow-to-warm-up* and *difficult*. Note that a large proportion of children do not appear to clearly fall into any of these categories. Note also that the development of temperament may be related to the development of attachment style in early infancy, and that temperament develops as a result of an interaction between genetic factors that influence temperament and the environment. The interactive nature of genetic and environmental factors is a common theme is current developmental psychology.

- There is stronger evidence that temperament is related to adult personality than there is that attachment style is related to adult personality. This is perhaps unsurprising, as temperament and adult personality are closer together in time. *Parenting style* appears to be closely related to all three measures of behaviour (attachment, temperament, personality).
- A number of risk factors have been identified for the development of specific disorders (especially schizophrenia and depression). Nevertheless, the presence of several risk factors may not result in apparent disorder: *resilience*, or *invulnerability*, refers to this apparent resistance to environmental adversity. In contrast, certain individuals appear highly *vulnerable* to environmental risk factors. While the mechanism underlying this is unclear it is likely to be accounted for in part by the coping style adopted by the individual.

COGNITIVE DEVELOPMENT

Piaget's model

Jean Piaget (1896–1980) suggested a genetic epistemological model of cognitive development, derived almost entirely from observations of his own children (leading to subsequent criticism and making interpretation of the original difficult because of the discursive, non-experimental reporting style). The most important insight (and about the only conclusion still universally accepted) is that the thinking of children is qualitatively different rather than quantitatively different to that of adults. That is, children think differently to adults rather than less or poorly in comparison.

The term 'genetic epistemology' is used because the development of knowledge (epistemology) is the result of pre-programmed behaviours (genetic) that lead to consequences such that knowledge of the world arises through the organisation and understanding of these consequences. That is, knowledge and cognitive development depends on the interaction of the child with the physical and social worlds. The cognitive development of the child progresses in stages, with completion of one stage being a necessary condition before the next stage can begin. Although there is a rough time scale for each stage of development these are highly flexible, and consequently it is the order of the stages that is of primary importance.

Certain key concepts are important:

- *Egocentrism* refers to the child's initial inability to distinguish his or her own perspective from that of others.

- *Schemes* or *schemas* are patterns of knowledge and behaviour, from playing with toys to understanding how to behave in a restaurant.
- *Operations* are logical procedures allowing mental manipulation of thoughts, number, concepts, etc. and are not readily displayed in behaviour.
- *Assimilation* refers to the attempts made by the child to understand novel situations with reference to existing schemas.
- *Accommodation* refers to the ability to modify existing schemas in order to understand novel situations (which cannot be understood by a process of assimilation).

The stages of Piagetian theory are (in order, with rough time scale):

- *Sensorimotor* (0 to 18th months). The infant behaves in a reflexive way, learning basic stimulus–response relationships (i.e. cause and effect). Gradually, the infant learns to differentiate the self from the external world, and that objects remain when not perceived. No understanding of temporal relationships is evident.
- *Preoperational* or *symbolic* (18th month to 7th year). The child uses symbolic schemas (imaginary play, drawing, etc.) but is still highly egocentric (which gradually declines as the ability to understand alternative perspectives develops). Perception influences judgement (e.g. tall glasses contain 'more' water than squat ones, even when water is poured from one to the other).
- *Concrete operational* (7th to 11th year). Logical thought appears, for example conservation of quantity (tall glasses no longer contain 'more' water). Mental or physical actions can be reversed, especially reasoning with number and quantity. There is understanding, for example, that size remains the same as distance increase (i.e. less influence of perceptual factors). Egocentrism disappears.
- *Formal operational* (11th year onwards). Reasoning and thought can be entirely verbal or logical and self-reflective. Complex logical operations are possible ($A > B, B > C, A?C$). The child can reason from other perspectives and understand abstract concepts (good, bad, justice, etc.). Entire systems of belief develop, as well as complex self-identity.

In fact, the formal operational stage is very rarely reached by 11 years, and there is evidence that a significant proportion of adults rarely or never think in such a way, unless constrained to do so by the task. Note that those investigating cognitive development tend to think in formal operational terms (because of the educational system they have passed through), and that may account for overestimation of the incidence of such thought. There is also evidence that style of thinking is in part influenced by cultural factors; for example, egocentrism remains highly salient in Western cultures.

Thought and communication

The developmental stage that a child is at, according to Piagetian theory, has implications for how communication will proceed between the child and an adult.

In the *preoperational stage*, the child displays a considerable growth in linguistic skills, moving from single word utterances, through short sentences, to competent, if unsophisticated, language use. Towards the end of the preoperational stage the development of linguistic pragmatics (i.e. rules for the *appropriate* use of language, rather than simply how to form sentences) takes place. This is a largely social skill and depends to an extent on the understanding and appreciation of alternative perspectives. As such, children early in the preoperational stage fail to grasp such conversational rules as when it is appropriate to say certain things. For example, a child early in the preoperational stage may not appreciate that what he is saying is of little interest to the other party. Indirect questions, hints, sarcasm, and so on all require a certain degree of cognitive development before these skills can be learned. The most noticeable change towards the end of the preoperational stage is the development of politeness in the linguistic competence of these children.

Communication in the *concrete operational stage* develops primarily in parallel with the reduction and disappearance of the egocentrism that characterises younger children. Specifically, the ability to take alternative perspectives becomes fully developed, so that these children are able to say what other individuals do and do not know. Perhaps of most relevance to the child is the extent to which this development facilitates the persuasive communication which the child can use: preoperational children tend to simply reiterate crude requests, while concrete operational children use more devious forms of persuasion which take into account the attitudes and desires of the (usually) adult to whom the request is directed. The other striking development is the development of *humour*, reflecting a certain degree of cognitive development. In particular, the incongruity central to many jokes requires the ability to take alternative perspectives in order for this to engender humour.

Finally, the *formal operational* stage, in the context of communication, represents the final development of the social skills that must be allied to linguistic ability. An increasing level of subtlety is evident in requests and persuasion, and the use of pragmatics appears. Questions may be asked of those connected to the source of information rather than the source of information itself (e.g. asking a mutual friend about someone else's opinion). The sophistication of the humour used also increases, in particular becoming more subtle, for example the use of satire and irony rather than simple sarcasm. The understanding of unfamiliar words also develops, so that specific definition is not required and may be inferred from the context of the sentence in which the new word is found.

Limitations in the communicative ability of children and adolescents, therefore, stem from the cognitive development evident at different ages. This clearly has implications for understanding children of different ages, and also for conveying information in a way that is likely to be understood. As the capacity for abstraction develops, egocentrism correspondingly declines, while the social skills of communication (pragmatics) develop:

- Spoken language becomes complex and more directed at achieving goals in a social context.
- Abstract concepts become more readily understood.
- Written communication develops as the needs/perspective of the reader can be appreciated.

Summary

- Piaget's model of cognitive development, while no longer universally accepted, remains the most influential model in the area. It is important to be aware of certain key concepts that underpin the model: *egocentrism*, *schemes*, *operations*, *assimilation* and *accommodation*. These represent the key mechanisms that allow the infant to progress through the distinct stages proposed by Piaget. An important feature of the model is that the infant must complete one stage before being able to continue to the next. One recent criticism is that this approach is excessively rigid and in reality the cognitive development of infants is more fluid.
- The stages of Piaget's theory are: *sensorimotor*, *preoperational*, *concrete operational* and *formal operational*. One should be aware of the characteristics of these stages and the rough ages at which the infant passes through them.
- *Linguistic ability* and *communicative skill* are closely related to Piagetian stage. In particular, the social rules of language, such as taking into account that the other party may not be interested in what is being said, require particular cognitive abilities such as the ascription of mental states to others. Given that language may be regarded as goal-directed behaviour carried out in a social context, the ability to understand abstract concepts is important.

LANGUAGE DEVELOPMENT

The development of language is a clear example of the interaction between innate behaviours in children and environmental influences. By acquiring language, the infant becomes able to send and receive highly complex strings of information. Note some definitions:

- *Phonemes* are basic units of sound which can be used to construct word sounds.
- *Morphemes* are made up of phonemes and are word or meaning units.
- *Syntax* is the structure of the sentence formation (i.e. grammar).
- *Semantics* is the meaning of a sentence or utterance.
- *Pragmatics* is the relationship between the words used and the (social) uses of them.

Language may be described by a complex set of syntactic rules, and the acquisition of language may be regarded as the acquisition of these rules. However, these rules are usually not consciously accessible to language speakers in any detail, even though we are highly competent at generating sentences within these rules and identifying errors. Chomsky (1993) has suggested that there exists a common underlying structure to all languages (universal grammar) related to genetic factors that enable language acquisition (language acquisition device).

Similar to Piaget's theory of cognitive development, language acquisition proceeds through stages, with widely varying rates. Some evidence that rate of language acquisition is related to subsequent intelligence.

- *First year.* Pre-linguistic stage, consisting of infant noises (crying, cooing, etc.). Infants initially learn to categorise sounds made by others and, after 3–4 months begin to 'babble', i.e. strings of phonemes. By the end of the first year, the range of phonemes uttered reduces to those specific to native language. First words spoken by end of first year.
- *Second year.* One or two dozen words spoken by the 18th month, but in no order. By the end of the second year, words are paired in a rigid order, reflecting knowledge gained from interactions with other objects ('my ball'). Vocabulary increasing rapidly (c.300 words – very crude estimate).
- *Third year.* Some sense of syntax/grammar emerges, with utterances becoming longer to accommodate this. Sometimes grammatical rules overgeneralised, for example always adding 's' to pluralise words (e.g. 'mouses', 'sheeps'). Words learned very rapidly.
- *Fourth year.* Use of grammar broadly correct, but utterances/sentences very simple, and few syntactic devices are used in any single sentence. Understanding is greater than ability to generate sentences. Future tense begins to be used.
- *Fifth year.* Language begins to resemble adult language, including social rules (allowing others to speak, etc.). Several clauses included in sentences. Verbal thought becomes apparent, including awareness of own ability to use language.

Note that simple models of learning (e.g. operant conditioning) are insufficient to account for the richness of language and the speed at which it develops (cf. Chomsky). Certain critical periods for language development exist:

- First year of life crucial for differentiation of phonemes.
- Syntactic development over first few years important.

In particular, language deprivation in the child's early years leads to inhibition of language acquisition subsequently (although still possible, full competence is never achieved). There is some evidence from deaf children that similar principles apply to sign language acquisition.

Environmental influences

Given that language is used for communication, it is not surprising that language development relies on the use of language in a social context, learning relationships between objects, individuals, situations, etc. While cognitive development is necessary for the acquisition of language, it is not sufficient. Indeed, cognitive development appears to outstrip linguistic development, in particular in reference to the self, with the child often using his or her name all the time to refer to themselves. What is evident is that the child wishes to express certain meanings, and language is one way in which this may be done. In this sense, linguistic development should be regarded in a broader social context. That is, the child may wish to draw the mother's attention to an object, and this may be done in a variety of ways: glancing, pointing, grabbing motions will all achieve this. Language is yet another way in which such a meaning may be expressed, and has certain advantages over crude options such as grabbing. Therefore, language acquisition is one part of the development of communication skills, which continues to develop long after the basic elements of language are learned (i.e. social rules, schemas, etc.).

The social and environmental context within which language is learned is important: infants begin by distinguishing all phonemic forms and only later reduce these to those required within their native language. This effect is strong enough to make the correct pronunciation of foreign languages very difficult for most adults.

The complexity of a native language is also far greater than second languages learned later in life, where a 'basic variety' appears to be learned, without the same depth of syntactic complexity.

Finally, while there is evidence that early isolation from language impairs language acquisition in later life, it appears that this effect is greatest if there is social isolation also. While there are too few cases to draw general conclusions from, isolation from language but not from a rich social environment can later result in the learning of elementary linguistic skills. Isolation from both language and social stimulation, however, seems to result in far greater linguistic impairment.

Communicative competence

As mentioned earlier, what appears to be learned by infants is communicative competence, rather than specific linguistic competence. Instead, linguistic skills should be regarded as a sub-group of communication skills. This accounts for the very important influence of social context in the development of language.

It is important to keep clear the distinction between language and communication:

- A large number of species display degrees of *communicative competence*, but care should be taken in describing these as languages.
- While infants use single words quite early in life, at what point should this be described as language rather than communication?
- Non-verbal communication (body language) is a powerful means of communication, and appears to be closely related to language (Italians prevented from gesticulating make far more speech errors), so should this be regarded as component of language?
- Are systems of manual signing (e.g. American Sign Language; ASL) to be regarded as genuine languages? If so, do they also reflect a universal grammar (cf. Chomsky).

To conclude, an individual may be highly skilled at constructing sentences but lack the social skills to be able to talk freely with others, in particular with unfamiliar others. While linguistic ability is good, communicative ability is impaired, illustrating the partial dissociation of the two concepts.   *Autistic*

Summary

- Understanding certain key concepts is important: *phonemes* are basic sound units which, when combined, make up *morphemes*, representing word or meaning units; *syntax* refers to the structure of grammar of sentences, and *semantic* to the meaningful content of sentences. Language development, in a similar way to cognitive and moral development, has been characterised as progressing in stages. These stages are less clearly delineated than, for example, those in Piaget's theory; put simply, the initial stages are concerned with the acquisition of vocabulary and familiarisation with the basic rules of language structure, while later development is concerned with the application of language in a social context, as goal-directed behaviour. *Language deprivation* in early life results in semi-permanent linguistic deficit, with extent of this deficit being greater if the deprivation lasts longer.

- It is important to distinguish between *speaking* and *communication*. While it is clear that communication is a broader concept, it is perhaps less clear that an individual may have relatively well-developed linguistic skills but poor communication skills. Autistic individuals represent an example of this. Conversely, the ability to communicate effectively does not necessarily require the presence of linguistic ability, such as in certain animal species.

SOCIAL DEVELOPMENT

Development of social competence

The development of attachment behaviours and attachment styles corresponds to the development of an internal model (schema) of relationship formation and norms. This provides the basis for the development of social competence, but is by no means the end-point. A wide variety of rules exist for behaviour within any given society, and within contexts within that society. The formation of rules, schemas and scripts for behaviour in different contexts represents the basis of social competence.

Acceptance

The development of social competence is required for the individual to become part of a group, given the apparent fundamental need that humans have for group membership. The first stage of this is acceptance into the group, which is determined to a great extent by conformity; this appears to develop as the child's cognitive and social abilities develop. *Egocentrism*, and the inability to accommodate the desires and expectations of others in young children, results in a lack of conformity. By the end of the preoperational stage (see Piaget), at approximately 6–7 years, the child is better able to understand the social rules for behaviour. At this stage, children can become embarrassed by their parents in certain situations if specific rules for behaviour are broken. In keeping with the development of concrete operational thought, these rules tend to be rigid, becoming more flexible as the child's cognitive development continues.

Group formation

The crucial difference between peer groups and family groups is that in the former the individual will interact on an equal level with others in the group. The formation of peer groups (i.e. children playing together) appears to facilitate both social and cognitive development. What appears to benefit most from interaction with others in groups is the ability of the other to understand alternative perspectives and the development of rules for social behaviour (i.e. norms).

Co-operation

The development of social competence and norms for behaviour includes the emphasis placed on co-operation or competition. There appears to be a strong cultural influence here, with Western cultures being traditionally highly competitive and individualistic. The ingroup–outgroup biases found in minimal group experiments (see earlier) may be the result of the internalisation of social norms which promote competition rather than co-operation. Nevertheless, co-operation is required in some cases, and appears to be one of the major determinants of group behaviour. Co-operative behaviour appears in infants during the pre-operational stage of cognitive development, when children will be seen to play together and achieve joint goals or take on individual roles in a broader game.

Friendships

In early and middle childhood, as described above, the formation of groups and friendships is primarily required for the adequate development of cognitive and social skills. As the child matures, the importance of peer group attitudes and rules increases while the influence of the family group and parents decreases.

In *adolescence* the individual becomes aware that development is to an extent within one's own control, so that a contemporary is required to provide a model (or counterpoint) to the chosen personality. As such, the need for a 'best friend' becomes strong during this period. Several stages of friendship behaviour have been suggested during adolescence:

- Shared activity   –   the focus is on shared activities rather than self-identity formation.
- Shared identity   –   emotional and intellectual features of others become important.
- Individuality   –   differences and unique abilities in others begin to be appreciated.

Isolation and rejection

Low self-esteem seems to be closely related to isolation and rejection of indi-viduals by others. Low self-esteem is related to a lack of social skills and a sense of awkwardness when interacting with others, and with further con-sequences such as a lack of initiative in making friendships and an unwill-ingness to take part in group activities. (See the discussion of Erikson's (1968) model of the development of self-identity for a more detailed discussion.) Note that self-esteem develops relatively early in childhood, and continues to have an influence on social development through childhood to adulthood.

The factors determining isolation and rejection are not solely individu-alistic, however: the dynamics of group formation and behaviour indicates that any individual perceived as belonging to a minority (i.e. an outgroup) will be rejected by the ingroup. In this case, the direction of causation is reversed, with rejection resulting in a lowering of self-esteem.

Popularity

Friendships and group membership also influences what is regarded as desirable by the child; in particular, popularity and social acceptability becomes of prime importance. In any given group of young children cer-tain individuals will stand out as being particularly popular, while con-versely there will also be a few peripheral figures who do not feature strongly in the internal dynamics of the group.

Children in school classes asked who they would like to sit near, work with, etc. tend to reflect this structure by naming only a few members of the class, such that graphical representations may be created from the chil-dren's answers, with dots representing individuals and arrows from these representing which of the other members of the group are regarded as pop-ular. On the basis of these studies popular children are suggested to be:

- Good-looking.
- Athletic (in males).
- Friendly.
- Extraverted.
- Socially competent.
- Intelligent.

The difficulty with research of this type – and in particular because of the role of the group in facilitating the development of certain components of popularity – is that it is difficult to determine the direction of causation: does extraversion result in popularity, or does popularity result in extra-version?

There is also a strong relationship between popularity and *leadership*; indeed, popular children tend to be the informal leaders of group activities. One factor that is apparent in leaders rather than those who are simply popular is aggression, although this is highly controlled aggression, used primarily to reinforce the leader's position when required. Uncontrolled aggression, in contrast, is associated with unpopularity.

Summary

- As should be clear from other sections, the development of social competence and social skills is integral to the development of moral and communicative ability. One particularly strong motive force in social behaviour is the tendency to form *groups*, frequently on the basis of weak or non-existent criteria other than some perceived common ground, however insignificant (cf. the minimal group paradigm).
- While the dynamics of group formation and friendship formation are relatively constant throughout the lifespan, the nature of *friendships* varies somewhat with age. This is related to the role friendships play in the development of social competence, in particular the need to make comparisons and assess what is accepted within a particular social context.
- One should be aware of the similarities and differences between *acquaintances* and friends. While both may serve an important and similar function in social development, friends tend to have a greater impact on the development of internalised social norms.

MORAL DEVELOPMENT

Kohlberg's theory

Kohlberg (1981) suggests a stage model of moral development, comparable in some ways to Piaget's model of cognitive development:

- Preconventional morality
  Level 1 – avoidance of punishment
  Level 2 – acquisition of rewards
- Conventional morality
  Level 3 – acquisition of social reward (approval)/avoidance of disapproval
  Level 4 – defined by concrete rules, laws, etc.

- Postconventional morality
  Level 5 – defined by the 'public good', a social contract
  Level 6 – individual moral code, abstract personal ethics

This model was derived from subjects' responses to a series of ethical dilemmas presented to them, with the answers being analysed in detail. There is some correspondence between moral 'level' and age, but even in adults the proportion of people who respond in a way that corresponds with the highest level of morality is small. Kohlberg himself suggested that this level would be achieved by very few and would be evident only in those regarded as paradigms of morality. In early and middle childhood, the vast majority of moral judgements are made with reference to punishment and rewards, with this gradually shifting towards social rather than physical punishment and reward. It is not until *adolescence* that any concept of the 'public good' becomes apparent.

Unfortunately, the correlation between moral development as assessed by Kohlberg's model and actual behaviour is quite weak. This weakness is probably due to the emphasis that the model places on abstract reasoning and the description of moral behaviour, as opposed to its actual perform-ance. The advances through the levels of morality with age may simply be the result of an increased awareness of and ability to describe moral rules, without necessarily being related to any desire to follow these.

Social perspective-taking

The ability to form a detached opinion from another person's perspective, or from a general 'social' perspective represents a significant advance in the cognitive and moral development of the individual. This requires a strong sense of personal identity, an understanding of the independence of the thoughts and actions of others (i.e. cognitive development), and an under-standing that morality is not simply defined by one's own desires and cor-responding rewards and punishments (i.e. moral development). Consequently, it is unsurprising that Kohlberg's level at which an under-standing of social norms for moral behaviour becomes apparent corre-sponds (roughly) with the development of concrete operational thought and a corresponding decline in egocentrism.

The ability to reason from perspective other than one's own, however, is distinct from the desire to act in a moral way (see above: criticisms of Kohlberg). Social perspective-taking is a largely cognitive ability that may be applied to moral dilemmas, so that the stages of Kohlberg's theory may only represent an increasing ability to reason from perspectives other than one's own (rather than any actual development of personal morality).

Summary

- Kohlberg's theory of moral development is a stage theory with three distinct stages of morality: *preconventional, conventional,* and *postconventional*). Development does proceed over time but not in as rigid a way a proposed by, say, Piaget's model of cognitive development. Note that a significant proportion of adults never reach the stage of postconventional morality (reserved by Kohlberg himself for 'moral giants').
- There is some correspondence between moral development and *cognitive development*, given that more abstract moral principles require the ability to appreciate the perspective of others.

DEVELOPMENT OF FEARS

Childhood and adolescence

Very young infants are characterised by a relative lack of fear in most situations. While certain situations do elicit a fear response in newborns (such as the visual cliff, where infants placed near a perceived ledge will show increased heart rate and breathing rate), most do not. Separation from the mother, for example, or the presence of strangers only induces anxiety after about the 6th month (see Attachment). It appears, then, that while some situations are innately fearful, the majority of fear responses (indeed, some components of the fear response itself) must be learned.

- 0–6th months: fear of only very specific environmental conditions (dark, height, etc.).
- 6th–12th months: development of stranger anxiety and separation anxiety (attachment).
- Early childhood: vicarious acquisition of fears from attachment figures (e.g. mother); learning of fear responses (classical and operant conditioning).
- Adolescence: relative strength of learning processes decreases, still greater than in adults; many normal fears decline over time.

As a general rule, younger children tend to be more receptive to learning processes, and therefore are more likely to develop fear responses (e.g. a young child, who was presented with an initially neutral object, a rabbit, paired with a loud noise, so that a fear of rabbits developed).

Note that while the fear response is a biological response, including physiological elements (e.g. increased heart rate) as well as behavioural elements, some elements are learned by observation of others, in particular the use of language to communicate fear.

Note also that some fears/phobias exist which are specific to childhood. An example is 'school phobia', which is probably best regarded as a pathological case of separation anxiety. There is some debate over the value of this classification, and the term is rarely used. Some fears (e.g. of the dark) are common in childhood, and usually decline over time.

Aetiological and maintenance mechanisms

Learning theory models of the development and maintenance of fears and phobias have proved successful. Several mechanisms are likely to act in parallel:

Classical conditioning

The association of a neutral object with an unpleasant noise, shock, etc. will result in the reaction to the noise, say, resulting when exposed to the neutral stimulus alone. That is, fears are suggested to be the result of the association of neutral objects with fear-evoking objects. *Stimulus preparedness* refers to the fact that individuals appear to develop fears of certain objects more readily than others (e.g. snakes), and it is suggested that there may be a genetic component to this readiness. (See the earlier discussion under learning theory for more detail.)

While valuable in understanding the development and maintenance of phobias, this model is also appropriate in understanding normal fear. In particular, infants appear to learn fearful behaviour from the observation of attachment figures, in particular the mother. This may be described as a form of vicarious classical conditioning, or as social learning theory. Note that the two models are not exclusive.

Operant conditioning

While of less relevance in understanding the development of fears, operant conditioning models provide some insight into the *maintenance* of fears (or, more properly, fear responses). Given that escape or avoidance behaviour results in the reduction of fear or the prevention of it altogether, this behaviour will be reinforced. Therefore, once a fear has become established, normal fear behaviour (e.g. escape) will serve to maintain the fear. This has implications for the treatment of fears (again, see section on learning theory).

Note that all learning processes are more powerful in early childhood, and this corresponds with the fact that most fears develop early in life and are sustained through it. Adults rarely develop new fears except in extreme circumstances (e.g. post-traumatic stress disorder).

Summary

- Certain fears appear to be largely innate (heights, dark, etc.), and there may be an evolutionary component to this. Other fears appear to be learned, in particular vicariously through observation of attachment figures. In this case there is some evidence for the '*preparedness*' of certain stimuli, whereby fears appear to form more readily for, for example, snakes rather than curtains. Again, an evolutionary components has been suggested to account for this phenomenon.
- Different models of learning are of relevance in understanding the development and *maintenance* of fears: classical conditioning, operant conditioning and social learning/modelling theories have all been proposed. All are useful in understanding different aspects of the development of fears.

SEXUAL DEVELOPMENT

Physical sexual development takes place primarily over a 3- to 5-year period, and is characterised by rapid physical growth and the more gradual development of sexual characteristics (facial hair and deeper voice in males, for example). There is substantial variation in the time of onset of puberty and the rate of development, although in the majority of cases development is complete by the 16th or 17th year.

This physical development is accompanied by increases in emotionality and, importantly, changes in self-identity, self-esteem and social relationships. While there is some evidence that this is related in part to the hormonal changes associated with sexual development, such a link is likely to be weak. In particular, sexual development significantly earlier or later than one's peers can be distressing. This interacts with sex, so that late-maturing boys show greatest distress (compared with early-maturing boys), while the reverse pattern is true of girls. It should be noted that any behavioural and emotional problems that exist during puberty and adolescence usually disappear with age.

Sexual identity

The development of personal identity is a central feature of adolescence, and is discussed in more detail in a later section (see p. 159). A significant component, most closely related to sexual development, however, is the development of sexual identity. Specifically, sexual identity refers to the elements of self-identity, self-perception, etc. which pertain to sexual preference (see below). It is more general than simply the delineation of sexual preference, however, in that it also encompasses the extent to and way in which the individual's sexuality is expressed and portrayed to others. As such, certain behavioural and psychological characteristics may be described as masculine or feminine, with any individual (regardless of sex) displaying both masculine and feminine features. Several theories have suggested ways in which sexual identity develops:

- *Psychoanalytic* (Freud): the sex drive is initially directed towards the father (in females) and is blocked by the mother, so that the child identifies with the mother in order to achieve the father (or substitute), leading to appropriate gender roles.
  - the basic mechanism of Freudian theory is identification.
  - incestuous love/sex drive is repressed.
  - the Oedipus or Electra complex results.
  - culminates in c. 5th year.
  - identification leads to the adoption of gender role.
- Social learning: cultural and societal forces model the behaviour of the child from birth, as well as the behaviour of others towards the child (e.g. girls play with dolls, are dressed in pink [!] etc.), leading to the development of sexual and gender identity.
  - behaviour, and therefore self-identity, is socially learned.
  - learning proceeds through reward, punishment and observation.
  - physical development, sexual characteristics, etc. are of minor importance.
  - child gradually learns appropriate social behaviour, which is internalised.
  - part of this includes the internalisation of appropriate gender behaviour.
- Cognitive development: as the cognitive development of the child progresses, there is an increasing awareness of the self, including important elements of the self-concept such as 'she' or 'he', which is gradually incorporated into the child's understanding.
  - sex/gender concepts are poorly understood in young children.
  - <5th year sex is identified by clothing, hair length, etc.
  - identity is fluid; changing a simple characteristic is enough (e.g. zebra – stripes = horse).
  - c. 5th year clearer understanding of concepts develops.
  - this results in awareness of own sex and corresponding sexual identity/role.

It is important to realise that, again, these alternative explanations are not exclusive. Furthermore, similar processes (especially social learning) may account for the development of other elements of personal identity and self-image/concept, such as socioeconomic status, ethnic group, etc.

Sexual preference

Sexual preference, simply, is the preferred sex of one's partner, and is a behavioural index defined by the usual sex of the partner. It is a relatively recent term, used to distinguish between *subjective sexuality*, which is rarely polarised as either heterosexual or homosexual, and actual *sexual behaviour*, which usually is. *Sexual orientation* comprises several components, including attraction, behaviour, affection, etc. As a result, the classification of individuals as either heterosexual, or homosexual, or bisexual is overly simplistic. There is substantial current interest in the extent to which sexual orientation and sexual preference is innate or learned.

To date, any evidence in either direction is equivocal and no firm conclusions may be stated confidently. Such research has been more successful at disconfirming hypotheses, so that the following conclusions have been supported to some degree (disconfirming common hypotheses and some popular beliefs):

- Sexual preference is established relatively early, usually before puberty and adolescence, even if the individual is uncomfortable with this identity, and precedes sexual activity.
- The nature of the first sexual encounter appears unimportant, with homosexuals being as likely as heterosexuals to have had a first sexual encounter with a partner of the opposite sex.
- Homosexuals appear to have participated in less sexually stereotyped behaviour as children, so that a lack of conformity appears to be associated with subsequent homosexuality.
- Parental relationships appear to be of little importance, undermining psychoanalytic theories of the development of sexual preference.

Studies investigating the genetic contribution to sexual preference have suggested that there is a genetic component to sexuality. For example, increasing genetic similarity is related to an increasing correspondence of sexual behaviour (for a more detailed description of the methodologies used, see the earlier section on frameworks for conceptualising development, p. 119). However, as in the case of intelligence or personality, care must be taken in interpreting these results, given the complex nature of genotype–phenotype interactions. It is possible that certain genetically determined characteristics result in certain behaviour being more or less likely which, in this society, is likely to result in a certain self-identity being developed (i.e. more or less stereotypically masculine), which is likely to be reinforced externally.

Summary

- One should distinguish between *physical* and *psychological* sexual development. While the former, to a large extent, drives the latter, it is the latter where there is greater scope for individual variation and a description of the causal factors more difficult. Psychological sexual development corresponds broadly to the development of a distinct sexual identity.
- Three broad theoretical positions exist for understanding the development of sexual identity and preference: *psychoanalytic* theories emphasise the role of basic drives and desires; *social learning* theories focus on the role of social and cultural norms; *cognitive developmental* theories suggest that cognitive development results in an increasing awareness of the self, including sexual identity.
- The development of sexual identity includes the development of *sexual preferences*. Evidence suggests that preference is established in early life with parental influence being minimal. Such research is clearly controversial and care must be taken in interpreting results.

ADOLESCENCE

Pubertal changes

Pubertal changes are those associated with the development of the sex organs such that these enable reproduction. These changes are more obvious in females at menarche (first menstrual period), while in males the changes are more gradual. Certain physical changes are apparent, in particular in males, such as the development of facial hair, deeper voice, etc. The point at which puberty ends is difficult to define, and there is no clear value in attempting to set a period for this, in particular given the wide variation across individuals in onset and rate of development. Note the distinction between:

- Primary sexual changes   – specifically of the sex organs.
- Secondary sexual changes – of other physical characteristics (facial hair).

It is *secondary sexual changes* that are most noticeable: males grow significantly in size, and body proportions also change (the shoulders broaden, etc.), while in females breasts develop. There is also some evidence that cognitive differences between males and females emerge at puberty, with males being more likely to take spatial and mathematical subjects at school while females are more likely to take verbal and literary subjects. Evidence for these differences is somewhat controversial, and the effect seems to be largely determined by social pressures. Nevertheless, it has been suggested that there are sex-related differences in brain organisation.

Note that these physical changes are accompanied by important developments in *self-image*. For example, drawings of the self change noticeably over the first menstrual period in females, even though this is a very short period of time, incorporating far more stereotypically feminine characteristics (not necessarily reflecting actual physical changes).

Task mastery

Physical and cognitive changes associated with puberty and adolescence allow for the development of new abilities. This period is also associated with a high degree of social development, in particular the development of sexual relationships (see above, Sexual identity). Social development is also accelerated as result of the stronger peer relationships that develop, providing a set of group and attitude norms that become internalised. Self-esteem and personal achievements are also highly correlated. This physical, cognitive and social development results in the achievement of autonomy:

* Behavioural autonomy – the ability to select activities and friends independently.
* Emotional autonomy – increasing independence from family members.
* Value autonomy – value and beliefs determined more by peers than family.

In summary, adolescence requires mastery of two developmental tasks:

* Development and acceptance of adult sexuality.
* Development and acceptance of social identity (and autonomy).

Conflict

It is a common public stereotype that *adolescence* and *puberty* are associated with conflict with authority figures, in particular parents and teachers. While there is some support for this stereotype, it appears that such behaviour is largely culturally determined. For example, in Western cultures childhood is regarded as unique, and the transition to adulthood is an important one, while at the same time parental control is high. This results in the characteristic desire of adolescent children to assert their individuality and achieve independence. In contrast, there is some evidence that the distinction between childhood and adulthood is less clear in some cultures (e.g. Chinese) and the degree of parental control sought is less, and that this corresponds to a relatively conflict-free adolescence.

Not only does conflict appear to be largely generated by social norms (rather than, say, excessive emotionality related to hormonal changes; see below), but it is also a function of changes in self-image and self-esteem. Development into an adult is associated with increased self-esteem and confidence, and as such a greater ability to assert oneself (as opposed to simply a desire to do so). Finally, the stereotype (as is the nature of stereotypes) of adolescent conflict is too general, and there is a large proportion of individuals who pass through adolescence without any major conflict or turmoil.

Affective stability

It has been repeatedly suggested that the hormonal and other physiological changes associated with adolescence result in some degree of emotional instability. While there is some evidence that emotionality is higher during adolescence, this effect is in fact far weaker than has been proposed. Moreover, the effect is as likely to be the result of social conflict as physiological factors. Indeed, the notion of adolescent affective lability has existed in literature at least as far back as the 18th century, suggesting a strong role for social construction. While there is undoubtedly a degree of conflict associated with adolescence (above), this is more likely to be the result of the changing self-image and self-esteem of the individual, rather than any affective instability. Moreover, those adolescents who do experience a high degree of emotional instability are likely to continue to display this in adulthood.

Normal and abnormal development

Adolescence should be regarded as a developmental stage characterised by significant physical and psychosocial changes. While the notion of adolescence and puberty as a time of great turmoil is largely unfounded, these changes nevertheless require a substantial degree of adaptation on the part of the adolescent. As outlined above, the majority of these changes, while initiated by physical changes and the psychological and social consequences of these, are related to self-image and self-expression. Normal development will be associated with changes in a variety of areas:

- Values and belief patterns.
- Social behaviour patterns.
- Sexual behaviour patterns.
- Cognitive abilities (independent, logical and abstract thought).
- Physical abilities.
- Self-esteem.
- Self-image/self-concept.

While there is evidence that some adolescents do experience distress and turmoil, this appears to be abnormal and is associated with similar affective instability in later life. Adequate adjustment to the demands of adolescence is a very strong predictor of successful adaptation in adulthood.

Adolescent conduct and behavioural problems are strongly associated with *criminal behaviour*, both in adolescence and later in adulthood. This is in part culturally influenced, in that in cultures where pubertal and adolescent turmoil is regarded as normal, the incidence of adolescent criminality is far higher than in cultures where the emphasis on adolescence is far less.

Summary

- Physical change in adolescence is marked, and there are correspondingly marked psychological changes, in particular in social and sexual identity. Note the distinction between *primary* and *secondary* sexual changes.
- Physical, cognitive and social development results in the accomplishment of specific tasks (task mastery). In particular the *adolescent* must develop sexually and socially and, most importantly, be comfortable with and accept these changes.
- Changes in self-image, social identity and so on may result in a degree of conflict between the adolescent and, usually, authority figures. This, however, is less common than popularly believed. While some have suggested that emotionality is elevated during adolescence as a result of hormonal fluctuations the evidence for this is weak.
- Abnormal adolescent development is usually characterised by an inability to accept sexual and social changes associated with this period, or by development in this area being impaired in some way.

ADAPTATIONS IN ADULT LIFE

Adulthood should not be regarded as the end-point of development, and adaptation proceeds throughout life. Certain specific adaptations are common to most individuals, each representing a significant change in lifestyle and an attendant change in self-identity, responsibility, etc. These may include:

- the decision to choose a partner for life;
- whether or not to have children; and
- choosing an occupation.

Pairing

It is likely that the first significant change in the lifestyle of an adult will be the formation of a romantic relationship that is intended to be permanent. Although an increasing number of couples do not marry, the majority still do. Regardless of the exact nature of the relationship with the partner certain features are common. The following factors appear to be important in the development of romantic relationships:

- Attractiveness.
- Common attitudes.
- Emotional stability.

Note that there is an association between marriage (i.e. the existence of a permanent partner) and health, both physical and mental. A happy and stable relationship is a protective factor, while unhappy relationships have been associated with poorer immune function, greater depression, etc.

Parenting

The transition to parenthood affects the behaviour of both the mother and the father, and may change the quality of the marital relationship (for better or worse). Mothers tend to become more sexually stereotyped, engaging in more feminine behaviours and less masculine behaviours. In contrast, fathers become less sexually stereotyped, with a relative increase in feminine behaviour becoming apparent. The factors that may influence the quality of the marital relationship include:

- Relative reduction in income.
- Potential absolute reduction in income.
- Sleep disturbance.
- Reduction in privacy.

While these factors suggest that the transition to parenthood should have negative consequences for the marriage, there is contrasting evidence that intimacy and affection increases between the marital partners, so that the stress of parenthood is moderated. In general parenthood is likely to be more stressful if:

- The parents are young.
- The birth takes place before marriage.
- The relationship has existed for a long period prior to the birth.

Note also that the temperament of the child (see earlier) will also have an impact on how stressful the transition to parenthood is, with difficult children representing a greater challenge.

Illness

Illness may be regarded as a relatively common but nevertheless serious source of stress in individuals. Beyond the physical effects of the illness the individual will be required to appraise their condition and, in adults, typically include both current concerns (e.g. loss of income) and concerns about the future.

Note also that the *nature of illness* that individuals have to cope with and adapt to, changes with age. As the individual ages, illness becomes more common and chronic illness becomes more likely. The illnesses suffered are also likely to become more serious and debilitating (e.g. stroke). In the case of chronic illness it has been suggested that individuals pass through several stages of adjustment:

- Shock   – the initial phase: bewilderment and a sense of detachment are common.
- Encounter – characterised by grief, despair and depression.
- Retreat   – denial appears, either of the illness or its implications.
- Intrusion – gradually the individual comes to terms with the illness and adapts.

This model has been criticised for being excessively rigid and prescriptive, but there is some evidence that at least a large proportion of individuals reacts to the diagnosis of chronic illness in roughly the way described above.

Bereavement and loss

While bereavement is generally used to refer to the loss of a relative, close friend, loved one, etc., it may also be more generally used to refer to other forms of loss, such as limb amputation or loss of a job. The common feature of these cases is that a considerable degree of adjustment is required after the loss, although of course there will be variation in severity and reaction across individuals. Commonly, bereaved individuals:

- see their doctor more often;
- are more likely to die themselves in the 6 months following the bereavement;
- become preoccupied with the object or individual that has been lost;
- show loss of appetite and general apathy; and/or
- exhibit signs of denial.

These responses to bereavement are common and should be regarded as normal, provided that the individual eventually adjusts to the loss. Several factors have been associated with poor adjustment:

- Lower socioeconomic status.
- Several concurrent, stressful life events.
- Self-blame.
- Severe depression.
- Lack of forewarning and preparation.

While in some cases adjustment to the loss may be difficult and lengthy, the majority of individuals eventually do adapt effectively.

Summary

- Adaptations in adult life are characterised by a requirement of the individual to interact in specific, socially defined ways, with others. A perfect example is the search for a partner and subsequent parenting. While one may choose not to take such decisions it is usual, and socially acceptable, to follow a fairly clearly defined path through life, punctuated by periods of adaptation (marriage, parenthood, bereavement, death, for example).
- Note that no definitive list of the adaptations required in adulthood exists, but in general one should consider major events that require a significant change in lifestyle of the individual. In such cases there will be role played by self-image, self-esteem and so on, and also by others (e.g. social support).

PREGNANCY AND CHILDBIRTH

The nine months of pregnancy represent a gradual build up to the stresses of childbirth and parenthood, while also representing a stressful episode itself.

Physiological stresses

The physical changes associated with pregnancy are (perhaps paradoxically) not regarded as particularly feminine, in particular by women themselves. The increase in weight, and the hormonal (especially progesterone and oestrogen) and dietary changes that result from pregnancy, represent a significant source of physiological stress, with consequent problems such as back pain and morning sickness. The physiological consequences also contribute to a great extent to the feeling of unattractiveness common in many pregnant women.

At the time of birth the most important consideration of the mother is the pain associated with childbirth. Relaxation and focused-attention techniques do allow significantly improved tolerance of pain, while other methods of childbirth have broader objectives such as the maintenance of contact between the mother and child.

Psychological stresses

The onset of pregnancy will have consequences not only for the mother but also for the father. For example, the preoccupation of the mother with the foetus may result in feelings of alienation and separation in the father. Although there is no reason why sexual contact should be reduced during pregnancy it commonly is, and there is some evidence that sexual behaviour during pregnancy is related to the ease of labour. Several stereotypes and attitudes exist towards pregnancy:

- *Pregnancy as illness*: the substantial medical intervention in births may result in a conception that the birth is a medical (rather than natural) process.
- *Pregnancy as crisis*: the professional consequences of pregnancy for employed women may be substantial, in particular if the pregnancy is unplanned or unexpected.
- *Pregnancy as a task*: there is substantial pressure, in some case, from other family members for a couple to begin a family, which may not correspond to the couple's wishes.

These stereotypes and attitudes tend to be most strong during the first pregnancy; contact with the realities of pregnancy and childbirth tend to engender a more realistic and mature attitude in mothers having a second child. However, this may also have negative consequences if the events during pregnancy are highly aversive, such as prolonged labour, so that the mother may expect a difficult labour again even if this is relatively unlikely.

Anxiety is a common feature of pregnant mothers, and may be focused on several potential risks or outcomes, such as:

- possible handicap of the child;
- preoccupation with cleanliness;
- own abilities as a mother;
- financial consequences of a child; and/or
- risk of miscarriage.

While some degree of anxiety is perhaps to be expected, there is evidence that excessive stress during pregnancy may influence foetal development in several ways, and has also been shown to be related to the risk of miscarriage and low birth weight.

It should also be realised that the incidence of miscarriage is significant and results in very strong grief reactions from both parents, especially the mother, being associated with subsequent depression for several weeks or months following the event.

Summary

- One should distinguish between the *physiological* and *psychological stresses* of pregnancy and childbirth, although these clearly interact. Post-natal depression, for example, is likely to include a strong physiological (i.e. hormonal) component.
- Specific social stereotypes contribute to the stress of pregnancy and childbirth (for example, the pathologisation of pregnancy).
- A degree of *anxiety* is normal in pregnant mothers (and, indeed, in the fathers), generated by a variety of potential negative outcomes or consequences (financial burden, doubt in one's ability to act as a good parent, etc.).

DEVELOPMENT OF PERSONAL IDENTITY

Erikson suggests a stage model of psychosocial and personal development, with each stage being characterised by a particular crisis that the individual must overcome in order to develop.

Stage	Crisis	Favourable outcome
1st year	Trust/Mistrust	Trust and sense of security (attachment).
2nd year	Autonomy/Self-doubt	Self-control, self-efficacy.
3rd–5th years	Initiative/Guilt	Confidence in own ability to act/initiate.

6th–13th years	Competence/Inferiority	Competence in social and intellectual skills.
Adolescence	Identity/Confusion	Development of self-identity.
Adulthood	Intimacy/Isolation	Commitment to others, career, etc.
Middle-age	Generativity/Stagnation	Concern beyond self to family, society, future.
Later life	Integrity/Despair	Sense of satisfaction, completion.

While the results detailed above represent favourable outcomes, the result of each psychosocial crisis may not in fact be favourable, resulting in anxiety, insecurity, loneliness, etc. The ability to face each crisis depends on a large extent to the outcome of the previous crisis, so that a child who develops secure attachments and a strong sense of self-control in early life will be well prepared to face future challenges and crises.

Various social identities

Social identities derive largely from the membership of groups, although these groups need not be explicit (such as membership of a football team) and may be more implicit (such as recognition of oneself as belonging to a certain socioeconomic class). As such, individuals will possess a number of social identities that may overlap and, in some cases, conflict.

Group memberships appears to be a fundamental need (see earlier discussion) such that individuals will very rapidly regard themselves as belonging to a group, even on the basis of random and meaningless criteria, and display a preference for other members of the group as a result. Note that:

- Individual identity (self-concept) depends to a large extent on social identities.
- Intergroup comparisons contribute to self-esteem.
- The need for a positive self-concept results in intergroup prejudice and bias.

The question 'Who am I?', asked of subjects and repeated several times, results in an interesting and insightful hierarchy of self-descriptions, many of which are related to social identities and group membership. This is influenced by cultural factors also, so that in Western cultures there is a bias towards individual characteristics while in Eastern cultures there is more emphasis on group membership.

Note also that social identities need not necessarily be related to group membership (although the majority are), and may instead relate to perceived relationships and interactions with other (e.g. a strong component of self-concept may be 'father').

Adaptations in adult life

Typical adaptations in adult life include the development of permanent romantic relationships, the birth of the first child, the onset of serious illness, and bereavement. These have been discussed in more detail previously. Nevertheless, the development of the individual, in particular social support, self-esteem and self-efficacy beliefs, will influence the degree to which the individual adapts to various life crises. Therefore, factors that influence the extent to which adaptations in adult life will be successful include:

- Self-esteem
- Self-efficacy
- Locus of control
- Attributional style
- Social support

Using Erikson's model of the development of personal identity it is clear that developmental experiences, in particular those in early and middle childhood, will influence the above factors, as well as directly influencing coping responses to stressful events. That is, an individual with a strong, coherent and positive sense of self will be better prepared to cope with major life events requiring adaptation.

The 'mid-life crisis' represents the generativity/stagnation crisis of middle adulthood suggested by Erikson. The proposal is that adults at this stage question their achievements to date, and what they will achieve in the remainder of their life. Priorities tend to be restructured, and greater emphasis is placed on the development of children, rather than the self. Nevertheless, the term 'crisis' is debatable as the evidence that individuals in middle adulthood are particularly distressed is weak. As such it is perhaps more valuable to examine specific crises (i.e. adaptations) separately, with middle adulthood simply representing a period when several of these are likely to occur close together (e.g. illness, children leaving home, etc.).

Summary

- The basic structure of Erikson's model of personal development is important, in particular the crises which characterise different stages of the model. For each of these there is a general favourable (or unfavourable) outcome. Note that these outcomes are appropriate at

different stages in the lifespan, and the model is therefore distinct in that it covers the entire lifespan, from birth to death. Concern for the future and society in general, for example, is appropriate by this model in middle age but inappropriate in adolescence, where personal development and self-identity is paramount.
- The stages of Erikson's model correspond to an extent to the different social roles adopted by individuals over the lifespan. For example, parenthood in adult life corresponds to the development, in Erikson's model, of a commitment to others. One should be aware of the correspondence between Eriksonian stages lifespan adaptations.

AGEING

Individual functioning and ageing

The physical, physiological and cognitive changes related to ageing result in corresponding changes in the individual's functioning. For example, speed of performance:

- generally becomes slower;
- is not uniform across tasks;
- is <10% between 20th year and 70th year for aimed movement;
- shows a c. 25% decline for simple sensorimotor decision tasks; and/or
- shows a c. 50% decline for complex sensorimotor decision tasks.

Sensory function, in particular vision and hearing, also declines. The most significant changes begin after the 40th year, when decline in function becomes much more rapid.

- Memory and learning
  - Learning of new skills declines.
  - Longer explicit recall also declines with age.
  - Some memory tasks show improvement (due to greater use of memory aids?).
- Personality
  - Erikson regards development through the lifespan as continual (see earlier section).
  - Norms for psychometric personality questionnaires (e.g. EPQ) change with age.
  - Individuals generally become less extravert and less neurotic.
  - Emotionality is more stable and easily controlled.
- Sexuality
  - Nature of sexual function changes greatly.

- Pleasure derived from intercourse often remains.
- Sexuality in the elderly often not socially accepted.
- Common misconception that elderly cannot (or should not) remain sexually active.

Social functioning and ageing

Social contact generally reduces with age. While this is in part due to a reduction in the number of friends, the changes in individual functioning (above) associated with age also lead to a reluctance or inability to maintain social contact.

- Social situations may be frightening if hearing, vision, etc. is impaired (e.g. busy streets).
- Difficulties in performing certain tasks required for social contact (e.g. walking to a bus stop).
- Society may not allow for the differences in individual functioning found in the elderly (i.e. objects, places, etc. are designed by the young and healthy, usually without consideration for the elderly).

Nevertheless, there are certain gains associated with age, such as reduced emotionality, which may allow certain losses to be compensated for. Selective optimisation with compensation may be used to refer to ability of individuals to:

- select appropriate and realistic goals;
- focus on goals of primary importance; and/or
- use alternative strategies to compensate for declining abilities (e.g. use of memory aids).

This conceptualisation is universal, although clearly the pattern of behaviour and compensation will vary widely across individuals.

Summary

- The normal ageing process has both physical and psychological consequences. The physical consequences are relatively straightforward, including a gradual decline in *sensorimotor ability*, *memory* and so on. Apparent improvements in certain types of memory with age may be ascribed to increasing use of memory aids.
- Psychological consequences of ageing include changes in the *sexual behaviour* of individuals. Note that this is primarily due to social norms rather than any decline in the desire for or pleasure derived from intercourse. Social contact also changes, as a consequence of a declining social network and an inability to perform certain social tasks as a result of physical changes.

DISABILITY AND PAIN

Disability

There are three important definitions required for a complete analysis of disability:

- *Impairment*: this refers to the actual problem (physical or mental), such as amputation of a limb or impaired mental function.
- *Disability*: as a result of the impairment, certain behaviours become restricted or impossible, for example walking.
- *Handicap*: the social consequences of disability include the embarrassment resulting from the impairment, or the reduced social contact.

In particular, the subjective meaning of an *impairment* will be very different across individuals, and be mediated by such factors as social support, self-efficacy beliefs, attributions, etc. This will also interact with situational variables, so that the impact of a leg amputation may be very different for an active, young individual compared to an elderly, relatively inactive individual. The medical assessment of severity will use very different criteria to those used by the patient.

Disability commonly results in difficulties in two social areas:

- *Employment*: there is substantial evidence that individuals with disabilities are less likely to obtain full-time employment.
- *Relationships*: self-image may become more negative as a consequence of disability, and the perception of others will also tend to be prejudiced.

The onset of disability, and in particular social difficulties associated with this, will tend to result in a loss of self-esteem, such that the incidence of depression and social withdrawal is relatively high in individuals with a disability, in particular if the onset of disability takes place in adulthood. This effect is greatest shortly after the onset of the disability, and it is suggested that the coping process associated with disability is broadly similar to that proposed for bereavement (and, indeed, loss generally).

The grief associated with a loss (e.g. disability) is complex:

- The response is stereotyped, in that the physical and psychological symptoms are broadly similar across individuals (sleep disturbance, eating disturbance, etc.).
- The response is the consequence of a specific, well-defined event, such as the onset of serious disability or the loss of a spouse.
- While some elements of the grief response may be adaptive in the short term, they may become maladaptive (e.g. apathy and withdrawal do not engender acceptance and coping).

Note that while the majority of research has focused on grief in humans, there is also evidence that other animals display similar behaviour, especially primates.

Chronic pain

Cultural models of pain tend to represent it as something which is transient; patients with persistent pain tend to develop complex psychological and behavioural problems associated with the difficulties in adjusting to pain that does not resolve. Chronic pain patients tend to show:

- Depression.
- Extreme inactivity.
- Social withdrawal.
- Loss of social contact.
- Loss of employment.
- Highly externalised locus of control beliefs.
- Very low self-efficacy beliefs.
- Catastrophising thoughts.

Operant conditioning models of chronic pain suggest that the behaviours displayed by chronic pain patients (NOT the pain itself) may be the result of learning processes. This may be regarded as a special case of 'sick role' behaviours. Three types of reinforcement are suggested to exist in the context of a patient with pain that does not resolve:

- Primary gain: interpersonal, psychological mechanism, reducing negative affect.
- Secondary gain: intrapersonal, environmental advantage supplied by behaviour.
- Tertiary gain: any advantage supplied by someone other than the patient.

Briefly, the behaviours typical of an individual in pain, such as inactivity and request for sympathy, medication, and so on, may result in positive and negative reinforcement (e.g. receiving sympathy, avoiding unpleasant work). If this persists for a sufficient period the behaviour becomes reinforced to such an extent that it becomes disabling. Note that this is not necessarily a conscious process, and the model specifically does NOT state that the patient's pain is the result of conditioning processes, simply the behaviour.

Treatment programmes based on this approach admit the patient to a unit and proceed to reverse the pattern of reinforcement, so that activity is positively reinforced. Although such programmes are highly selective, success rates are striking, with patients showing marked increases in activity levels and reductions in medication consumption. Reported pain decreases, even though this is not specifically targeted by the treatment.

Summary

- Note the distinctions between 'impairment', 'disability' and 'handicap', given that the three terms are frequently but mistakenly conflated. Note that any given disability will result in very different reactions across individuals and medical criteria used to assess disability often fail to take these individual differences into account.
- Psychological models of learning have proved fruitful in explaining the development and maintenance of specific behaviour in chronic pain patients. This model may be extended to include the behaviour of disabled individuals generally and may also have some application in understanding the behaviour of depressed patients. One should appreciate that the operant conditioning processes suggested to underlie certain behaviours are not conscious and behaviour change may occur automatically rather than being the conscious will of the individual (a common misconception).

DEATH AND DYING

There is an enormous amount of literature on the impact of a terminal prognosis, and the acceptance of death by individuals. As in most studies of loss, several stages have been suggested by, among others, Kubler-Ross (1969):

- *Denial*: the initial prognosis is not believed; this may recur as the individual adjusts.
- *Anger*: this may be directed towards care staff and relatives.
- *Bargaining*: the patient may attempt to gain better care by agreeing to behave well.
- *Depression*: grief is overt and shared between the patient and the family/friends.
- *Acceptance*: detachment and a sense of calm characterises the final stage.

As with most stage models of loss, a common criticism is that the stages are too prescriptive and need not occur in a set order. Denial, for example, tends to recur often through the coping and adjustment process. It is perhaps more valuable to understand the various reactions which are likely, but also that they may occur at any time and in any order.

There are three main consequences of terminal illness that the patient must adjust to:

- Worsening physical condition.
- Restriction of activity and substantial change in social circumstances.
- Realisation that life is nearly at an end.

The family and friends of the patient will also cope with and adjust to a terminal prognosis, and problems may arise if the adjustment of the family does not proceed as smoothly as that of the patient. For example, it is not uncommon for family members to continue to deny the impending death of the patient after the patient has come to terms with the prognosis.

Poor adjustment in the patient (such as excessive denial or dependence on others) has been shown to be related to more rapid decline. Patients who maintain high levels of social support and social interactions tend to be those who survive longest.

It is important to realise that dying is a protracted and complex social process, with death itself simply representing one point in this process that, for the family, does not even represent the end-point. The adjustment of the family and friends of the patient to the death may be greatly facilitated before the death by allowing substantial communication and intimacy. The control of pain, therefore, must be balanced against the reduction in communication that results from high dosages of pain medication.

Summary

- The frequently cited model of Kubler-Ross for death and dying consists of several stages through which the individual and the family must progress. An important feature of this model is that apparently *poor adaptation* to loss (denial, anger, etc.) are in fact necessary and normal stages of grieving. There are criticisms of the rigidity of this model.
- Be aware that death, dying and loss in general has implications beyond the individual concerned to the family and social network in general. There will be similarities and differences in the process of adaptation that characterises each, and conflict often arises when, for example, the family adjusts at a different rate to the individual (and is therefore at a different stage).

HUMAN DEVELOPMENT INDIVIDUAL STATEMENT QUESTIONS

1. Gender identity is morphological sex assigned at birth.
2. Gender identity is the sex in which the child is reared.
3. Gender identity is the child's own belief about his or her own sex.
4. Gender identity is defined by the preference of a sexual partner.
5. Gender identity is coded on the X chromosome.

6. Coping styles linked to vulnerability to psychiatric disorder have been described in terms of attribution theory.
7. Coping styles linked to vulnerability to psychiatric disorder have been described in terms of effort after meaning.
8. Coping styles linked to vulnerability to psychiatric disorder have been described in terms of learned helplessness.
9. Coping styles linked to vulnerability to psychiatric disorder have been described in terms of perceived inadequacy of social relationships.
10. Coping styles linked to vulnerability to psychiatric disorder have been described in terms of locus of control theory.

11. According to Piaget's theory of cognitive development, concrete operational thought indicates a psychotic process.
12. According to Piaget's theory of cognitive development, schemata can be modified by experience.
13. According to Piaget's theory of cognitive development, accommodation represents a compromise forced by reality testing.
14. According to Piaget's theory of cognitive development, the stage of formal operations is not entered before adolescence.
15. According to Piaget's theory of cognitive development, preoperational thought is magical in quality.

16. The depressive position is described by Bowlby as a phase in the reaction to loss.
17. Disorganisation is described by Bowlby as a phase in the reaction to loss.
18. Identification with the lost object is described by Bowlby as a phase in the reaction to loss.
19. Apathy is described by Bowlby as a phase in the reaction to loss.
20. Protest is described by Bowlby as a phase in the reaction to loss.

21. A lack of opportunities to form selective attachments is likely to result in indiscriminate friendliness towards strangers in later childhood.
22. A lack of opportunities to form selective attachments is likely to result in catastrophic reaction to failure in later childhood.
23. A lack of opportunities to form selective attachments is likely to result in antisocial behaviour in later childhood.
24. A lack of opportunities to form selective attachments is likely to result in separation anxiety in later childhood.

25. A lack of opportunities to form selective attachments is likely to result in attention-seeking behaviour in later childhood.

26. At the age of 2 years a typical child can draw a recognisable house.
27. At the age of 2 years a typical child uses the pronoun 'I'.
28. At the age of 2 years a typical child displays imaginative play with representational toys.
29. At the age of 2 years a typical child uses a knife and fork at table.
30. At the age of 2 years a typical child is dry by night.

31. With respect to adolescent development, rebellion against parental ethical values is virtually universal.
32. With respect to adolescent development, boys enter puberty earlier than girls.
33. With respect to adolescent development, body image disturbance is more common in girls than boys.
34. With respect to adolescent development, unstable personal identity is most likely when self-esteem is low.
35. With respect to adolescent development, fleeting ideas of reference are reported by about one-quarter of 15-year-olds.

36. In theories of motivation, Maslow's hierarchy of needs places self-actualisation above safety.
37. In theories of motivation, Mowrer distinguished between primary and secondary drives.
38. In theories of motivation, the relationship between arousal and learning can be represented graphically by a straight line.
39. In theories of motivation, the 'need for achievement' described by McClelland is linked with levels of aspiration.
40. In theories of motivation, incongruity within a familiar context is seen as stimulating competence.

41. Carl Gustav Jung described the unconscious as composed of both the personal unconscious and the collective unconscious.
42. Carl Gustav Jung emphasised that birth order played a key role in the development of personality styles of siblings.
43. Carl Gustav Jung was largely responsible for the humanistic school of psychology.
44. Carl Gustav Jung described universal images and concepts found repeatedly in mythologies of different cultures.
45. Carl Gustav Jung developed a schema for describing personality types according to three axes.

46. Biofeedback involves the system of reward and punishment based on the use of restricted diet in neurotic patients.
47. Biofeedback can modify cardiovascular function.
48. Biofeedback involves the transmission to subjects of information about biological function.

49. Biofeedback cannot be used without a good patient/therapist relationship.
50. Biofeedback is a useful method for reducing muscle tension.

51. Aversion therapy is based on the work of Pavlov.
52. Aversion therapy is exemplified by the use of disulfiram in alcoholics.
53. Aversion therapy is of proven use in the treatment of drug addicts.
54. Aversion therapy is of no use in the treatment of transvestitism.
55. Aversion therapy is useful in the treatment of sexual deviants.

56. Behavioural psychotherapeutic techniques include dichotomous thinking.
57. Behavioural psychotherapeutic techniques include response prevention.
58. Behavioural psychotherapeutic techniques include thought blocking.
59. Behavioural psychotherapeutic techniques include repression.
60. Behavioural psychotherapeutic techniques include implosion.

61. In behavioural psychotherapy, the patient's consent is not vital.
62. In behavioural psychotherapy, the measurement of progress is rarely possible.
63. In behavioural psychotherapy, modelling is of value in adults.
64. In behavioural psychotherapy, internal conflict is explored.
65. In behavioural psychotherapy, selective abstraction is of use in depression.

66. According to the tenets of behavioural psychopathology, neurotic symptoms are instances of learned maladaptive behaviour patterns.
67. According to the tenets of behavioural psychopathology, childhood fantasies are important in the genesis of neurosis.
68. According to the tenets of behavioural psychopathology, the underlying meaning of overt behaviour must be studied closely.
69. According to the tenets of behavioural psychopathology, the relationship between therapist and patient is critically important in treatment.
70. According to the tenets of behavioural psychopathology, maladaptive behaviour which persists must be undergoing reinforcement.

71. Systematic desensitisation is enhanced by massed learning.
72. Systematic desensitisation is enhanced by extinction.
73. Systematic desensitisation is enhanced by reciprocal inhibition.
74. Systematic desensitisation is enhanced by habituation.
75. Systematic desensitisation is enhanced by counter-conditioning.

76. Escape conditioning is involved in agoraphobia.
77. Avoidance conditioning is involved in agoraphobia.
78. Sensitisation is involved in agoraphobia.
79. Over-determination is involved in agoraphobia.
80. Implosion is involved in agoraphobia.

81. The cognitive model of anxiety includes selective abstraction.
82. The cognitive model of anxiety includes catastrophisation.
83. The cognitive model of anxiety includes hypovigilance.

84. The cognitive model of anxiety includes the fact that it only applies if intelligence is above average.
85. The cognitive model of anxiety includes abnormal thinking as an underlying process.

86. The behavioural assessment of obsessional behaviour includes asking patients about their mood.
87. The behavioural assessment of obsessional behaviour includes interviewing relatives.
88. The behavioural assessment of obsessional behaviour includes diary keeping.
89. The behavioural assessment of obsessional behaviour includes use of self-completed rating scales.
90. The behavioural assessment of obsessional behaviour includes asking the patient to approach feared situations.

91. In the behavioural formulation of phobias, identification is invoked.
92. In the behavioural formulation of phobias, preparedness is invoked.
93. In the behavioural formulation of phobias, catastrophic thinking is invoked.
94. In the behavioural formulation of phobias, avoidance learning is invoked.
95. In the behavioural formulation of phobias, incubation is invoked.

96. Piaget's concept of conservation refers to the inability of the child to alter his or her behaviour.
97. Piaget's concept of conservation is widely used in educational programmes.
98. Piaget's concept of conservation offers an explanation of excretory disorders in childhood.
99. Piaget's concept of conservation is closely related to Bateson's double bind.
100. Piaget's concept of conservation involves specified concepts of quantification.

101. Gender identity is morphological sex.
102. Gender identity is the sex a child is brought up to be.
103. Gender identity is the child's belief as to which sex he/she is.
104. Gender identity refers to sex-typed behaviour patterns.
105. Gender identity is always irreversible after 4 years of age.

106. Observations and experiments on maternal deprivation have been carried out by Bowlby.
107. Observations and experiments on maternal deprivation have been carried out by Jung.
108. Observations and experiments on maternal deprivation have been carried out by Malinowski.
109. Observations and experiments on maternal deprivation have been carried out by Piaget.
110. Observations and experiments on maternal deprivation have been carried out by Spitz.
111. Aetiological factors in failure of bonding include complicated childbirth.

112. Aetiological factors in failure of bonding include a teenage mother.
113. Aetiological factors in failure of bonding include maternal ambivalence about the pregnancy.
114. Aetiological factors in failure of bonding include an absent father.
115. Aetiological factors in failure of bonding include the newborn needing intensive care nursing and treatment.

116. Essential features of Piaget's theory of cognitive development include autonomy versus shame and doubt.
117. Essential features of Piaget's theory of cognitive development include basic trust versus mistrust.
118. Essential features of Piaget's theory of cognitive development include concrete operational.
119. Essential features of Piaget's theory of cognitive development include formal operational.
120. Essential features of Piaget's theory of cognitive development include sensorimotor.

121. Aggression in children is a relatively stable trait.
122. Regarding aggression in children, catharsis leads to decreased aggressive behaviour.
123. Aggression in children includes a genetic component.
124. Aggression in children may be reinforced by operant conditioning.
125. Aggression in children may be learned by modelling.

126. Gender identity depends on the chosen sexual partner.
127. Gender identity depends on morphological sex.
128. Gender identity depends on chromosomal sex.
129. Gender identity depends on the belief a person holds about his/her gender.
130. Gender identity depends on parents' influence (e.g. sex typing).

131. Regarding children aged under 2 years, if they are in day-care, they will have impaired maternal bonding.
132. Regarding children aged under 2 years, they may have more intense bonding with the father.
133. Regarding children aged under 2 years, a maternal substitute may adversely affect natural bonding with the child.
134. Regarding children age under 2 years, the amount of time spent with the child is of critical important in bonding.
135. Regarding children aged under 2 years, frequent visits from family is worse than total separation in children who have spent their life in hospital.

136. Most 1-year-old children are afraid of heights.
137. Most 1-year-old children are afraid of the dark.
138. Most 1-year-old children are afraid of animals.
139. Most 1-year-old children are afraid of loud noises.
140. Most 1-year-old children are afraid of strangers.

141. Attachment depends on parental reinforcement.
142. Attachment depends on eye contact.
143. Attachment may be increased if the mother is hostile.
144. Attachment does not occur with the father.
145. Attachment is related to behaviour in adolescence.

146. Bereavement does not increase mortality.
147. Bereavement increases the use of alcohol and tobacco.
148. Bereavement is associated with hallucinations.
149. Bereavement may be facilitated by 'forced mourning'.
150. Bereavement may produce 'morbid grief' as described by Lieberman (1979).

151. Behaviour therapy is associated with the experimental work of Skinner.
152. Behaviour therapy for severe depression lasts 30 hours on average.
153. Behaviour therapy may involve functional analysis.
154. Behaviour therapy may use a token economy.
155. Behaviour therapy is used in guided mourning.

156. In behavioural psychology, a coverant behaviour is a covert operant behaviour.
157. In behavioural psychology, Skinner's theories only describe observable non-verbal behaviours.
158. In behavioural psychology, the concept of shaping is associated with J.B. Watson.
159. In behavioural psychology, successive approximations can be used to teach procedures.
160. In behavioural psychology, a response is much harder to extinguish if it was acquired during continuous rather than partial reinforcement.

161. The stage of formal operations is a concept regarding the developing mind associated with Piaget.
162. Object constancy is a concept regarding the developing mind associated with Piaget.
163. Conservation of energy is a concept regarding the developing mind associated with Piaget.
164. Genetic epistemology is a concept regarding the developing mind associated with Piaget.
165. The two-factor theory of intelligence is a concept regarding the developing mind associated with Piaget.

ANSWERS

1.	F	45.	T	89.	T
2.	F	46.	F	90.	T
3.	T	47.	T	91.	F
4.	F	48.	T	92.	T
5.	F	49.	F	93.	F
6.	T	50.	T	94.	T
7.	F	51.	F	95.	F
8.	T	52.	T	96.	F
9.	F	53.	F	97.	T
10.	T	54.	T	98.	F
11.	F	55.	T	99.	F
12.	T	56.	F	100.	T
13.	T	57.	T	101.	F
14.	T	58.	F	102.	F
15.	T	59.	F	103.	T
16.	F	60.	T	104.	F
17.	T	61.	F	105.	F
18.	T	62.	F	106.	T
19.	F	63.	T	107.	F
20.	F	64.	F	108.	F
21.	T	65.	F	109.	F
22.	F	66.	T	110.	T
23.	T	67.	F	111.	T
24.	T	68.	F	112.	F
25.	F	69.	F	113.	T
26.	F	70.	T	114.	F
27.	T	71.	F	115.	T
28.	T	72.	F	116.	F
29.	F	73.	T	117.	F
30.	F	74.	T	118.	T
31.	F	75.	T	119.	T
32.	F	76.	T	120.	T
33.	T	77.	T	121.	T
34.	T	78.	T	122.	F
35.	T	79.	F	123.	T
36.	T	80.	F	124.	T
37.	T	81.	F	125.	T
38.	F	82.	T	126.	F
39.	T	83.	F	127.	F
40.	T	84.	F	128.	F
41.	T	85.	T	129.	T
42.	F	86.	F	130.	F
43.	F	87.	T	131.	F
44.	T	88.	T	132.	T

133.	F	144.	F	155.	T
134.	F	145.	T	156.	T
135.	F	146.	F	157.	F
136.	F	147.	T	158.	F
137.	F	148.	F	159.	T
138.	F	149.	T	160.	F
139.	T	150.	T	161.	T
140.	T	151.	T	162.	T
141.	T	152.	F	163.	F
142.	F	153.	T	164.	T
143.	T	154.	T	165.	F

Reading list

Cognitive psychology

Allport A. Visual attention. In: Posner MI (ed.) *Foundations of Cognitive Science*. Cambridge, MA: MIT Press, 1989.

Schachter DL. Memory. In: Posner MI (ed.) *Foundations of Cognitive Science*. Cambridge, MA: MIT Press, 1989.

Teasdale JD. Cognitive vulnerability to persistent depression. *Cognition and Emotion* 1988; 2: 247–60.

Williams JMG. The cognitive theory of depression revisited. In: Williams JMG (ed.) *The Psychological Treatment of Depression: A Guide to the Theory and Practice of Cognitive Behaviour Therapy*, 2nd edn. London: Routledge, 1992.

Developmental psychology

Dunn J, McGuire S. Sibling and peer relationships in childhood. *J Child Psychol Psychiatry* 1992; **33**: 67–105.

Hill P. Recent advances in selected aspects of adolescent development. *J Child Psychol Psychiatry* 1993; **34**: 69–99.

Prior, M. Childhood temperament. *J Child Psychol Psychiatry* 1992; **33**: 249–79.

Rutter M. Family and school influences on behavioural development. *J Child Psychol Psychiatry* 1985; **26**: 349–68.

Rutter M. Pathways from childhood to adult life. *J Child Psychol Psychiatry* 1989; **30**: 25–51.

Rutter M. Nature, nurture and psychopathology: a new look at an old topic. *Dev Psychopathol* 1991; **3**: 125–36.

Taylor E. Developmental neuropsychiatry. *J Child Psychol Psychiatry* 1991; **32**: 3–47.

Experimental psychology

Baddeley AD. Working memory. *Science* 1992; **255**: 556–9.

Burton AM, Young AW, Bruce V. *et al.* Understanding covert recognition. *Cognition* 1991; **39**: 129–66.

Duncan J, Humphreys GW. Visual search and stimulus similarity. *Psychol Rev* 1989; **96**: 433–58.

Gigerenzer G. From tools to theories: a heuristic of discovery in cognitive psychology. *Psychol Rev* 1991; **98**: 254–67.

Kelley CM, Jacoby LL. The construction of subjective experience: memory attributions. *Mind Language* 1990; **5**: 49–68.

Newell A. Precis of "Unified theories of cognition". *Behav Brain Sci* 1992; **15**: 425–92.

Posner MI, Petersen SE. The attention system of the human brain. *Annu Rev Neurosci* 1990; **13**: 25–42.

Schachter DL. Understanding implicit memory: a cognitive neuroscience approach. *Am Psychol* 1992; **47**: 559–69.

Treisman A. Features and objects: the 14th Bartlett Memorial Lecture. *Q J Exp Psychol* 1988; **40A**: 201–37.

Interpersonal psychology

Shea SC, Mezzich JE. Contemporary psychiatric interviewing: new directions for training. *Psychiatry* 1988; **51**: 385–97.

Watts FN. Strategies of clinical listening. *Br J Med Psychol* 1983; **56**: 113–23.

Neuropsychology

Dalla Barba G. Confabulation: knowledge and recollective experience. *Cogn Neuropsychol* 1993; **10**: 1–20.

Ellis HD, Young AW. Accounting for delusional misidentifications. *Br J Psychiatry* 1990; **157**: 239–48.

Funnell E, Sheridan J. Categories of knowledge? Unfamiliar aspects of living and non-living things. *Cogn Neuropsychol* 1992; **9**: 135–53.

Kopelman MD. Amnesia: organic and psychogenic. *Br J Psychiatry* 1987; **150**: 428–42.

Marshall JC, Halligan PW. Blindsight and insight in visuo-spatial neglect. *Nature* 1988; **336**: 766–7.

Schachter DL. Toward a cognitive neuropsychology of awareness: implicit knowledge and anosognosia. *J Clin Exp Neuropsychol* 1990; **12**: 155–78.

Social psychology

Hewstone M. *Introduction to Social Psychology: A European Perspective*. Oxford: Blackwell, 1988.

Sabini J. *Social Psychology*. New York: WW Norton, 1992.

Bibliography

Atkinson RL, Atkinson RC, Smith EE, Bem DJ, Nolen-Hoeksema S. *Hilgard's Introduction to Psychology.* Fort Worth, Texas: Harcourt Brace, 1996.

Buckley P, Bird J, Harrison G. *Examination Notes in Psychiatry.* Oxford: Butterworth-Heinemann, 1996.

Chomsky N. *Language and Thought.* Wakefield, Rhode Island: Moyer Bell, 1993.

Erikson EH. *Identity: Youth and Crisis.* New York: Norton, 1968.

Henderson M, Freeman CPL. A self-rating scale for bulimia: the BITE. *Br J Psychiatry* 1987; **150**: 18.

Kohlberg L. *The Meaning and Measurement of Moral Development.* Clark University: Heinz Werner Institute, 1981.

Kubler-Ross E. *On Death and Dying.* New York: Simon and Schuster, 1969.

Lieberman MA, Borman LD, and associates. *Self-help Groups for Coping with Crisis: Origins, Members, Processes, and Impact.* San Francisco: Josses-Bass, 1979.

Paykel ES. Scaling of life events. *Arch Gen Psychiatry* 1971; **25**: 340–7.

Piaget J. *The Child's Conception of the World.* New York: Harcourt, Brace Jovanovich, 1929.

Reber A. *Dictionary of Psychology.* New York: Penguin, 1985.

Roth EJ, Davidoff G, Haughton J, Ardner M. Functional assessment in spinal cord injury: a comparison of the Modified Barthel Index and the "adapted" Functional Independence Measure. *Clin Rehab* 1990; **4**(4): 277–85.

Rotter JB. Generalized expectancies for internal versus external control of reinforcement. *Psychological Monographs* 1966; **80**: 1–28.

Scarr S, McCartney K. How people make their own environments: a theory of genotype–environment interactions. *Child Dev* 1983; **54**: 424–35.

Tantam D, Birchwood M. (eds) *Seminars in Psychology and the Social Sciences.* London: Gaskell, 1994.

liberright

Index

abuse, intrafamilial, and child development, 136–7
acceptance, and social development, 149
accommodation, and Piaget's stage theory, 125, 142–3
achievement, need for, and motivation, 43, 44–5
active perception, 16–17, 19
addictive behaviours, learning theories for, 7–8
adolescence, 159–62
  affective stability, 161
  conflict with authority figures, 160–1
  normal and abnormal development, 161–2
  pubertal changes, 159–60
  task mastery, 160
adulthood, adaptations in, 162–5
adversities, early and late, and development, 123–4
affect
  in adolescence, 161
  and attachment behaviour, 129–30
affiliation, 70
ageing, 170–1
aggression, 83–6
  individual differences, 85
  media influences, 85
  theories of, 83–4
agnosia, and brain organisation, 97
alertness, 54–5
algorithms, 32–3
alternate form reliability, of tests, 101
altruism, 86–7, 88
amnesia, and brain organisation, 94
amnestic syndrome, 28
aphasia, and brain organisation, 95–6
arousal level, 54
  and motivation, 42

arousal theory, and aggression, 84, 86
Asch, S, and group behaviour, 77
assessment tools, 101–4
  criterion-referenced approaches, 104
  intelligence assessment, 106–9
  neuropsychological assessment, 109–12
  norm-referenced approaches, 103–4
  ratio scores, 103
  reliability of, 101–2
  scales, 102–3
  validity of, 102
assimilation, and Piaget's stage theory, 125, 142–3
attachment behaviour, 128–33
  and affect regulation, 129–30
  early separation, 131–2
  and emotional development, 129
  failure of development of, 132
  insecure attachment, 130–1
  maternal bonding, 132
  pattern of, 128–9
  and personal relationships, 130
  secure attachment, 130
  and temperament, 140–1
attention, 20–2, 23, 54
attitudes, 63–7
  and behaviour, 66–7
  and cognitive consistency, 66
  components, 63
  measurement of, 64–5
  and persuasion, 65–6
attribution theory, 71–2, 75
auditory system
  attention, 20–1
  perception see perception
autism
  and attachment behaviour, 132
  and theory of mind, 73, 75

autonomy, in adolescence, 160
avoidance conditioning, 9
awareness, levels of, 53–8
  alertness, 54–5
  arousal level, 54
  attention, 54
  and biorhythms, 56
  dreaming, 55
  hypnosis and suggestibility, 56–7
  levels of consciousness, 53–4
  meditation and trances, 57
  parasomnias, 55–6
  sleep, 55–6
  unconscious processing, 54

Baddeley, AD, working memory model,
    25, 29
behaviour, and attitudes, 66–7
behavioural treatments, 13
  and conditioning, 9–10
  and habituation, 10–11
  reciprocal inhibition, 10
bereavement, 135–6, 164–5
biorhythms, 56
blindsight, 97
brain organisation, 93–9
  experimental methods, 93
  frontal lobe functions, 98
  language, 94–6
  memory, 94
  perception, 96–7
  visuospatial ability, 97–8
Broca's area, and language, 94–6

Cannon–Baird theory, of emotion, 46,
    48
chaining, and behavioural treatments,
    10–11
childbirth, stresses of, 165–7
childhood fear, 154–5
Chomsky, N
  language development, 145–7
  linguistics and interpersonal
      communication, 73–4
chronic pain, 173–4
chunking, and short-term memory, 25–6
circadian rhythms, 56
classical conditioning, 4
  and fear development, 155
cognitive appraisal theory, 46
cognitive consistency, 66
  and motivation, 43, 44–5
cognitive development, 142–5
  communication skills, 144–5

Piaget's stage theory, 124–5, 142–3,
    145
  and sexual identity development, 157
cognitive dissonance, 66, 67
  and motivation, 43
cognitive learning, 5–6
cohort studies, 126
communication skills
  and cognitive development, 144–5
  and linguistic skills, 148, 149
communicative competence, 148
communicative control, in relationships,
    79
concepts, 30–1, 33
conditioning
  and addictive behaviours, 7–8
  and behavioural treatments, 9–10
  classical conditioning, 4
  escape and avoidance conditioning, 9
  extinction, 6
  generalisation, 8
  incubation, 8
  and observational learning, 5
  operant conditioning, 4–5
  and phobias, 7–9
  secondary reinforcement, 8
  stimulus preparedness, 9
conflict, in adolescence, 160–1
conformity, and group behaviour, 77
consciousness, levels of, 53, 57
  altered states of consciousness, 56–7,
      58
  unconscious processing, 54
  see also awareness, levels of
control, locus of, 52
co-operative behaviours, 87–8
  and social development, 150
coping behaviour, and stress responses,
    51–2, 53
criterion-referenced assessment tools,
    104
critical periods in development, 121
  language development, 146–7
Cronbach's alpha, and reliability of tests,
    101–2
cross-sectional studies, 126
cueing, and behavioural treatments, 11
culture, influences on intelligence,
    108–9
curiosity, 41–2

death and dying, 174–5
declarative memory, 26, 29
deductive reasoning, 31–2, 33

deindividuation, and group behaviour, 78
dementia, 28
depression
    and learned helplessness, 52
    learning theories for, 7
    and retrieval of information from memory, 27
desensitisation, behavioural treatments, 10–11
development *see* human development
disability, 172–3
divorce, and child development, 136
dreaming, 55
drives and needs, and motivation *see* motivation
drug addiction, learning theories for, 7–8
dysfunctional family relationships, 134–5
dysgraphia, and brain organisation, 95–6
dyslexia, and brain organisation, 95–6

early separation, from attachment figure, 131–2
egocentrism, and Piaget's stage theory, 142–3
emotion, 45–8
    Cannon–Baird theory, 46
    cognitive appraisal theory, 46
    components of, 45
    differentiation of, 46–7
    frontal lobe functions, 98
    functions of, 47
    James–Lange theory, 45–6
    primary emotions, 47
    and retrieval of information from memory, 27
encoding, of information, 24, 29
enmeshment, in family relationships, 135
environmental factors
    early and late adversities, 123–4
    gene interactions, 122–3
        study methods, 127
    and language development, 147–8
    nature–nurture debate, 119–20
episodic memory, 26, 29
Erikson, EH, stage theory of personal development, 167–8
escape conditioning, 9
ethological theories, of aggression, 83, 86
exchange theory, and helping behaviour, 87
executive functions, and frontal lobes, 98
explicit memory, 26, 29
extinction, and conditioning, 6, 13

extrinsic theories of motivation, 40, 44
Eysenck Personality Questionnaire, 34

family relationships, 133–8
    bereavement, 135–6
    distorted family function, 134–5
    divorce, 136
    intrafamilial abuse, 136–7
    non-orthodox structures, 137–8
    parenting styles, 133–4
fears
    development of, 154–6
    see also phobias
fight or flight response, 48–9
figure–ground differentiation, 14
films, violence in, and aggression, 85
filtering of information
    and attention, 20–2
    and schizophrenia, 22
forgetting, 26–7
Freud, S
    personality theories, 36
    sexual identity development theories, 157
friendship, 70–1, 75
    and social development, 150
frontal lobe functions, 98, 99
frustration–aggression hypothesis, 83, 86
fugue, memory impairment in, 28

general adaptation syndrome, 48–9
general factor of intelligence (g), 105–6, 109
generalisation, 8
genetic epistemological model, 124–5, 142–3, 145
genetic factors
    environmental interactions with, 122–3
        study methods, 127
    in nature–nurture debate, 119–20
    and sexual preference, 158–9
Gibson, JJ, and active perception, 16–17
group behaviour
    and leadership, 77–8, 79
    and personal identity, 168–9
    and social development
        acceptance, 149
        co-operation, 150
        isolation and rejection, 151
        peer group formation, 150
        popularity, 151–2
    see also intergroup behaviour
groupthink, 78

habituation, and behavioural treatments,
    10–11, 13
hallucinations, 17
handicap, definition, 172
Heider, F, attribution theory, 71–2
helping behaviour, 86–7, 88
    and co-operation, 87–8
heritability, 120
heuristics, 32–3
higher mental functions, and frontal
    lobes, 98
homeostasis, and motivation, 40–1, 44
hostility, between groups, 81
human development
    adolescence, 159–62
    adulthood, adaptations in, 162–5
    ageing, 170–1
    attachment behaviour see attachment
        behaviour
    and chronic pain, 173–4
    cognitive development see cognitive
        development
    concepts in, 119–26
        early and late adversities, 123–4
        gene–environment interactions,
            122–3
        maturational tasks, 121
        maturity, 122
        nature and nurture, 119–20
        psychoanalytic theories, 124
        social learning theory, 124
        stage theories, 120–1
    death and dying, 174–5
    and disability, 172–3
    family relationships see family
        relationships
    fear response, 154–6
    language development see language,
        development of
    methodologies in, 126–8
    moral development, 152–4
    personal identity, 167–70
    pregnancy and childbirth, 165–7
    sexual development, 156–9
    social development see social
        development
    temperament see temperament
humanistic theories of personality, 37, 39
    Q-sort technique, 38–9
hypnosis, 56–7
hypothalamus, and homeostasis, 41

illness, adjustments to, 164
illusions, 17

impairment, definition, 172
implicit memory, 26, 29
incubation, and conditioning, 8
inductive reasoning, 31–2, 33
infants, attachment behaviour see
    attachment behaviour
information processing, 19–23
    attention, 20–2
    encoding, 24
    and schizophrenia, 22
ingroup, definition, 80
insecure attachment behaviour, 130–1
instrumental conditioning see operant
    conditioning
intelligence, 105–9
    components of, 105–6
    cultural influences, 108–9
    definitions, 105
    measurement of, 106–9
intelligence quotient (IQ), 106–7
inter-rater reliability, of tests, 101–2
interactionist approaches, to personality,
    37–8, 39
intergroup behaviour, 80–2
    hostility, 81
    prejudice, 80
    and social identity, 82
    stereotypes, 80–1
    see also group behaviour
interpersonal psychology, 69–75
    affiliation, 70
    attribution theory, 71–2
    friendship, 70–1
    language, 73–4
    person perception, 69–70
    social behaviour, 72–3
    theory of mind, 73
intrafamilial abuse, and child
    development, 136–7
intrinsic theories of motivation see
    motivation
IQ (intelligence quotient), 106–7
isolation, and social development, 151

James–Lange theory, of emotion, 45–6,
    48

Kohlberg, L, moral development theory,
    152–3
Kubler-Ross, E, model of death and
    dying, 174–5

language
    and brain organisation, 94–6, 99

and cognitive development, 144–5
development of, 145–9
  acquisition of language, 145–7
  communicative competence, 148
  environmental influences, 147–8
and interpersonal communication,
  73–4
and thought, 30
law of effect, and operant conditioning,
  4–5
leadership, 75–9
  characteristics of leaders, 75–6
  and group behaviour
    conformity, 77
    deindividuation, 78
    groupthink, 78
    polarisation, 77–8
  and popularity, 152
  power and obedience, 77
  social influence, 76
  social power, 76
learned helplessness, 52
  and depression, 7–8
learned resourcefulness, 52
learning theory, 3–13
  and addictive behaviours, 7–8
  and behavioural treatments, 9–10
  classical conditioning, 4
  cognitive learning, 5–6
  and depression, 7
  escape and avoidance conditioning, 9
  extinction, 6
  and fear development, 155–6
  generalisation, 8
  habituation, 10–11
  incubation, 8
  observational learning, 12
  operant conditioning, 4–5
  and phobias, 7
  punishment, 12
  reciprocal inhibition, 10
  reinforcement, 6–7
  reinforcement schedules, 11–12
  secondary reinforcement, 8
  stimulus preparedness, 9
levels of awareness see awareness, levels of
life events, and stress responses, 49–50
Likert scales, for attitude assessment, 64,
  67
linguistics, and interpersonal
  communication, 73–4
locus of control, and stress responses, 52
long-term memory, 23–4, 28–9
  forgetting, 26–7

organisation of, 26
retrieval, 25
storage, 24–5
longitudinal studies, 126–7
loss, adjustments to, 164–5
  death and dying, 174–5
  disability, 172–3
  and family relationships, 135–6

marriage, 163
Maslow, A
  hierarchy of needs, 44, 45
  humanistic theories of personality, 37
maternal bonding, and attachment
  behaviour, 132
maturational tasks, 121, 125
maturity, 122
media, influences on aggression, 85
meditation, 57
memory, 23–9
  and brain organisation, 94, 99
  chunking, 25–6
  disorders of, 28
  encoding, 24
  forgetting, 26–7
  models of, 23–4
  organisation of long-term memory, 26
  retrieval, 25, 27–8
  storage, 24–5
  working memory, 25
methodologies
  in psychological assessment see
    assessment tools
  in studies of development, 126–8
    cohort studies, 126
    cross-sectional studies, 126
    genetic / environmental influences,
      127
    longitudinal studies of individuals,
      126–7
Milgram, S, and obedience, 77
minimal group experiments, 81
modelling see observational learning
moral development
  Kohlberg's theory, 152–3
  social perspective-taking, 153
morphemes, definition, 146
motivation, 40–5
  and arousal level, 42
  and cognitive consistency, 43
  curiosity, 41–2
  extrinsic theories, 40
  and homeostasis, 40–1
    hypothalamic systems, 41

motivation – *contd*
  intrinsic theories, 41
  Maslow's hierarchy of needs, 44
  need for achievement, 43
  needs and drives, 40

nature and nurture, 119–20, 125
need–drive models of motivation *see*
    motivation
need for achievement, and motivation,
    43, 44–5
neuropsychological assessment, 109–12
neuropsychology, 93–9
  experimental methods, 93
  frontal lobe functions, 98
  language, 94–6
  memory, 94
  perception, 96–7
  visuospatial ability, 97–8
nomothetic theories of personality, 34–5,
    39
norm-referenced assessment tools, 103–4

obedience, and leadership, 77
object constancy, 14–15
observational learning, 5
  and aggression, 83
  optimal conditions for, 12
operant conditioning, 4–5
  and aggression, 83, 86
  and fear development, 155–6
operations, and Piaget's stage theory,
    142–3
outgroup, definition, 80
overprotection, in family relationships,
    135

pain, chronic, 173–4
parasomnias, 55–6
parenting
  styles of, 133–4
  transition to parenthood, 163–4
Pavlovian conditioning, 4
peer groups, and social development, 150
perception, 13–19
  active perception, 16–17
  and brain organisation, 96–7, 99
  development of, 17–18
  disorders of, 17
  figure–ground differentiation, 14
  object constancy, 14–15
  perceptual phenomena, 15–16
  principles of, 13–14
  set, 15

person perception, 69–70, 74
personal construct theory of personality,
    35–6, 39
  repertory grid test, 38
personal identity
  adaptations in adulthood, 169
  social identities, 168–9
  stage model of development of, 68–9,
    167–8
personality, 34–9
  assessment tools, 38–9
  humanistic theories, 37
  interactionist approaches, 37–8
  nomothetic theories, 34
  personal construct theory, 35–6
  psychoanalytic theories, 36
  radiographic theories, 34
  and temperament, 140–1, 142
  trait theories, 34–5
  type A behaviour, and stress responses,
    51
  type theories, 34–5
persuasion, and attitude change, 65–6, 67
phenotype
  gene–environment interactions, 122–3
    study methods, 127
  and nature–nurture debate, 119–20
phobias
  behavioural treatments, 9–11
  learning theories for, 7–9
  see also fears
phonemes, definition, 146
physical abuse, and child development,
    136–7
physiological stress response, 48–9, 53
Piaget, J, stage theory of cognitive
    development, 124–5, 142–3, 145
polarisation, and group behaviour, 77–8
popularity, and social development,
    151–2
power, and leadership, 77
pragmatics
  definition, 146
  and interpersonal communication,
    73–4
preconscious processing, 54
pregnancy, stresses of, 165–7
prejudice, 80
preparedness, 9, 155
primary emotions, 47
primary memory *see* short-term memory
problem-solving, methods, 32–3
procedural memory, 26, 29
prosocial behaviour, 86–8

prototypes, 30, 33
    and problem solving, 32–3
psychoanalytic theories
    of development, 124
    of personality, 36, 39
    of sexual identity development, 157
psycholinguistics, and interpersonal
    communication, 73–4
psychometric assessment *see* assessment
    tools
puberty, 159–60
punishment, 12

Q-sort technique, for personality
    assessment, 38–9

radiographic theories of personality, 34,
    39
    humanistic theories, 37
    personal construct theory, 35–6
    psychoanalytic theories, 36
ratio scores, in psychological assessment,
    103
reasoning, 31–2, 33
reciprocal inhibition, and behavioural
    treatments, 10
reinforcement
    and conditioning, 4–5, 6–7, 13
    schedules for, 11–12
    secondary reinforcers, 8
rejection
    in family relationships, 135
    and social development, 151
relationships, with others
    in adolescence, 160–1
    in adulthood, 163
    and attachment behaviour of infant,
        130
    family relationships *see* family
        relationships
reliability, of tests, 101–2
repertory grid, for personality
    assessment, 38
resilience
    to stress, 50–1
    and temperament, 141, 142
retrieval, of information from memory,
    25, 27–8, 29
Rogers, C, humanistic theories of
    personality, 37
romantic relationships, 163

scales, for psychological assessment,
    102–3, 104

schemas
    and Piaget's stage theory, 125, 142–3
    and retrieval of information from
        memory, 27–8, 29
schizophrenia, information processing
    in, 22
secondary memory *see* long-term
    memory
secondary reinforcement, and
    conditioning, 8
secure attachment behaviour, 130
self-concept, 68–9
self-esteem, 68
    and social development, 151
self-image, 68
self-recognition, development of, 68–9
semantic differential scales, for attitude
    assessment, 64–5, 67
semantic memory, 26, 29
semantics, definition, 146
sensation, and perception, 13–14, 18
sensory perception *see* perception
set, perceptual, 15
sexual abuse, and child development,
    136–7
sexual development
    sexual identity, 156–8
    sexual preference, 158–9
shaping, and behavioural treatments, 11
short-term memory, 23–4, 28–9
    chunking, 25–6
    encoding, 24
    retrieval, 25
    working memory, 25
single-parent families, 137–8
sleep
    deprivation of, 56
    dreaming, 55
    parasomnias, 55–6
    stages of, 55, 57–8
social behaviour, 72–3
social development, 149–52
    acceptance, 149
    in adolescence, 160–1
    co-operation, 150
    friendships, 150
    isolation and rejection, 151
    peer group formation, 150
    popularity, 151–2
    social competence, 149
social environment, and language
    development, 147–8
social exchange theory, and helping
    behaviour, 87

social identity
    and group membership, 82
    and personal identity, 168–9
social influence, 76, 79
social learning theory
    of aggression, 83, 86
    and development, 124
    of sexual identity development, 157
social perspective, and moral
        development, 153
social power, 76, 79
Social Readjustment Rating Scale, 49–50
somatosensory perception, and brain
        organisation, 97–8
spatial neglect, and brain organisation,
        97
speech, and brain organisation, 94–6
split-half reliability, of tests, 101–2
stage theories
    of development, 120–1, 125
    of language development, 146–7,
        148–9
    of personal identity development,
        167–8
    Piaget's theory of cognitive
        development, 124–5, 142–3, 145
states of awareness see awareness, levels
        of
stereotypes
    and intergroup behaviour, 80–1
    and social behaviour, 72–3
stimulus preparedness, 9, 155
storage, of information in memory, 24–5,
        29
stress, 48–53
    coping behaviour, 51–2
    learned helplessness / learned
        resourcefulness, 52
    and locus of control, 52
    physiological aspects, 48–9
    psychological reactions, 49
    situational factors, 49–50
    and type A behaviour, 51
    vulnerability and invulnerability to,
        50–1
subconscious processing, 54
suggestibility, and hypnosis, 56–7
syntax, definition, 146

task mastery, in adolescence, 160

television, violence on, and aggression,
        85
temperament, 138–42
    and child–parent relationships, 138–9
    and personality, 140–1
    types of, 139–40
    vulnerability and resilience, 141
terminal illness, 174–5
test–retest reliability, of tests, 101
tests in psychological assessment see
        assessment tools
thalamic theory, of emotion, 46, 48
theory of mind, and developmental
        disorders, 73
Thorndike, E, and operant conditioning,
        4–5
thought, 30–3
    concepts, 30–1
    and language, 30
    problem-solving, 32–3
    prototypes, 30
    reasoning, 31–2
Thurstone scales, for attitude assessment,
        64, 67
trait theories of personality, 34–5, 39
trance state, 57
twin studies, in human development, 127
type A behaviour, and stress responses,
        51
type theories of personality, 34–5, 39

unconscious processing, 54
unorthodox family structures, 137–8

validity, of psychological tests, 102
violence, media influences, 85
visual system
    attention, 20, 21–2
    perception see perception
visuospatial ability, and brain
        organisation, 97–8
vulnerability
    to stress, 50–1
    and temperament, 141, 142

Wernicke's area, and language, 94–6
working memory, 25, 29
    see also short-term memory

Yerkes–Dodson law, and motivation, 42